Athletic Ability and the Anatomy of Motion

Rolf Wirhed Fil lic

Lecturer in Biomechanics,
Department of Physical Education and Health,
Örebro University, Örebro, Sweden

Translated by A. M. Hermansson

Illustrated by Gamil Gabra, Stig Salander

New illustrations by Michael Courtney,
Bruce Hogarth, Gillian Murray

THIRD EDITION

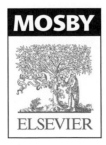

MOSBY

ELSEVIER

Edinburgh   London   New York   Oxford   Philadelphia   St Louis   Sydney   Toronto   2006

MOSBY
ELSEVIER

Originally published in Swedish as *Anatomi och rorelsclara inom idrotten (Samsprak Forlagsaktiebolag)* by Harpoon Publications AB, Örebro
Copyright © Rolf Wirhed, Harpoon Publications AB, 1982

First published in English by Wolfe Medical Publications, 1984
Copyright © Wolfe Medical Publications, 1984

Second edition published by Mosby, 1997
Copyright © Mosby, an imprint of Mosby International (a division of Times Mirror International Publishers Ltd), 1997

Third edition
© 2006, Elsevier Limited. All rights reserved.

First edition 1984
Second edition 1997
Third edition 2006

ISBN-13: 978-0-7234-3386-6
ISBN-10: 0 7234 3386 0

British Library Cataloguing in Publication Data
A catalogue record for this book is available from the British Library

Library of Congress Cataloging in Publication Data
A catalog record for this book is available from the Library of Congress

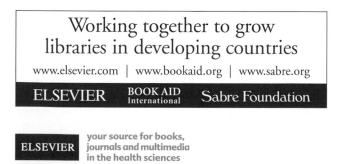

Working together to grow
libraries in developing countries

www.elsevier.com | www.bookaid.org | www.sabre.org

ELSEVIER   BOOK AID International   Sabre Foundation

ELSEVIER   your source for books, journals and multimedia in the health sciences
www.elsevierhealth.com

The publisher's policy is to use **paper manufactured from sustainable forests**

Printed in China

Contents

Preface

I have taught kinetics (or the theory of motion) at Örebro University of Physical Education for a number of years; this course deals with the mechanical laws that underlie exercise. Sportspeople are becoming increasingly interested in the application of these laws to sporting performance. Fitness instructors, for example, have become more aware of the need to teach correct movements in order to maximize the effectiveness of training and minimize the risk of injury. Exercises designed to prevent injury are now an important aspect of training for sport.

The first edition of *Athletic Ability and the Anatomy of Motion* was a response to the lack of suitable literature on the subject of 'biomechanics'. The book was designed to meet the need, expressed by sports leaders and sports associations, for a clear source of appropriate anatomical and mechanical knowledge. The second edition retained the structure of the first but was extensively revised and updated: discussion of the general characteristics of bones, joints and muscles was followed by coverage of the anatomy and function of different parts of the body. The main emphasis was placed on the analysis of movement, i.e. the biomechanical aspects of the exercises performed by sportspeople in training particular parts of the body. Different types of movement, such as take-off, rotation, flight and landing, were dealt with.

A section on muscle function, strength training and work capacity was added. This new edition contains additional material on strength training and numerous new illustrations, and has an expanded chapter on sports mechanics.

My own interest in this area was sparked by my enthusiasm for sport and by the training I received in atomic physics, which required a thorough knowledge of mechanics. I also studied anatomy in Uppsala so that I would better understand the mechanisms that allow the human body to perform various movements.

It is my hope that the readers of this book (including sports leaders, physical education teachers and physiotherapists) will find that examples contained in and ideas taken from this book will be of substantial practical value. The book may be used as a textbook for prospective physical education teachers, sports leaders and youth recreation leaders, and it may form the basis for adult education classes. Students of the natural sciences may find the book interesting as extra reading or be inspired by it when working on special projects. It is my hope that after having read this book, readers will have acquired a sound knowledge of the position and function of muscles, forces, momentum, the centre of gravity and the moment of inertia, and that they will find it easier to judge how to train. The general knowledge of anatomy and mechanics provided should enhance readers' ability to analyse and understand the sports in which they are interested. By carrying out the exercises and movements described, they will add to this a practical appreciation of kinetics; anatomy and kinetics should be experienced in practice – they are not solely theoretical concepts.

Finally, I would like to thank Neil Spurway for his considerable contribution to this edition.

Rolf Wirhed
Lecturer in Biomechanics
Department of Physical Education and Health
Örebro University
Örebro
Sweden

Chapter 1

General anatomy of bones, joints and muscles

A. The skeleton

The aim of this general section on the bones of the human body is to provide the reader with the basic knowledge needed to benefit from the literature on sports injuries, and also to aid in the analysis of how the bones react to the stresses and strains to which they are subjected in different training exercises.

The skeleton of the body is made up of a variety of bones, which are classified as follows:

1. Short bones – e.g. tarsals (bones of the ankle) and carpals (bones of the wrist).
2. Long bones – e.g. metacarpals (bones of the hand), ulna and radius (bones of the forearm) and femur (thigh bone).
3. Flat bones – e.g. bones of the skull, sternum (breastbone).

The process of bone formation is called ossification. The flat bones (e.g. the bones of the skull) are developed in one stage from connective tissue. This developmental process is called direct ossification (intramembranous ossification). The bones of the skull are not fully formed in the newborn baby. The areas of incomplete ossification, the so-called fontanelles, can be felt with the fingers. Most of the bones of the skeleton are formed by indirect ossification (intracartilaginous or endochondral ossification). A cartilaginous model of the future bone is developed in the embryo and is later resorbed and replaced by bone.

Short bones are formed by indirect ossification. The cells at the centre of the growing cartilaginous model die. The so-called osteoblasts (os = bone, blast = immature cell) migrate from the membrane that surrounds the cartilage (periosteum) to the spaces left by the wasted cells. These osteoblasts gradually change into bone cells (osteocytes). Not all the cartilage ossifies; some parts of it remain in the form of articular cartilage (Figure 1.1).

Articular fluid – which is found in the cavity of synovial joints – provides the articular cartilage with nourishment. Cells sitting in the inner layer

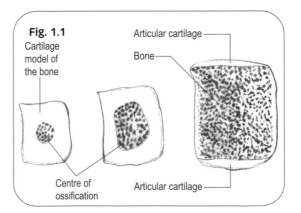

Fig. 1.1
Cartilage model of the bone

Articular cartilage

Bone

Centre of ossification

Articular cartilage

of the capsule that surrounds every joint produce the fluid. The blood vessels that lie inside the bone tissue, beneath the plates of articular cartilage, also supply nourishment to the cartilage. The nutrients diffuse through the cartilage cells (massaged into the cells by pressure on the joint) and are not transported through small blood vessels (capillaries). Thus, if the joints are subjected to suitable all-round stress during the formative years of childhood, they will be well supplied with nourishment. This in turn leads to a thickening of the cartilage, thereby providing better protection against the kind of injury caused by excessive stress. A joint that is not subjected to any kind of stress, or is not fully used in all possible directions, reacts in an opposite manner; that is, the cartilage thins down. When an athlete is limbering up before a special event the amount of articular fluid increases. The cartilage sucks up the fluid and becomes thicker for a couple of minutes. This protects the joint from being over stressed.

Figure 1.2 shows the epiphyseal cartilage (growth plates) situated at the proximal (towards the centre of the body) end of the

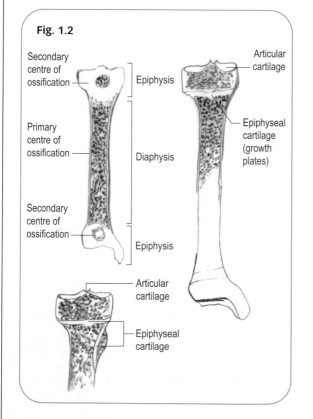

Fig. 1.2

Secondary centre of ossification

Epiphysis

Primary centre of ossification

Diaphysis

Secondary centre of ossification

Epiphysis

Articular cartilage

Epiphyseal cartilage

Articular cartilage

Epiphyseal cartilage (growth plates)

shaft of the tibia (shin bone) just beneath the insertion of the knee extensor muscles.

The long bones are also formed by indirect ossification, but here several so-called ossification centres can be found. In the formation of these bones, articular cartilage and epiphyseal cartilage are left between the shaft (diaphysis) and each extremity (epiphysis). The epiphyseal cartilage usually ossifies in the late teens or when a person is fully grown. The so-called epiphyseal cartilage can be located in a youth with the aid of an X-ray.

Pathological changes at the epiphyseal cartilage are often due to hormonal disturbances. They can also be a consequence of incorrectly loading or overloading the skeleton. Compared with the rest of the body the skeleton grows very quickly during the first few years of life and during adolescence. Athletically active young people should therefore refrain from *extreme* strength training during puberty. A good recommendation is that the child, while still undergoing the changes of puberty, should use only his or her own weight as a load when training. Thus, only the post-pubertal child should include weights and equipment in his or her strength-training routines.

A common complaint among children between the ages of 10 and 16 years is Osgood–Schlatters's disease. This condition results from excessive tension in the knee extensor's insertion on the small prominence of the tibia (tibial tuberosity). The epiphyseal cartilage is irritated and the ensuing growth may be accelerated. The enlargement can be seen with the naked eye when the affected leg is compared with the healthy one. The afflicted child may have difficulty in kneeling on hard surfaces.

Figure 1.3 shows the fully-grown bone in detail. Microscopically, small bone cells (osteocytes) lie embedded in a tissue consisting of collagen fibres (which are highly resistant to extension), inorganic salts (giving the bone its hardness) and organic salts (giving the bone its elasticity). The ratio between the inorganic and organic salts is 1:1 at birth, but changes to 7:1 by the time the body is 60–70 years old. This explains the skeleton's elasticity in youth and its brittleness in old age. Also shown in Figure 1.3 is the arrangement of bone cells in concentric circular layers around a

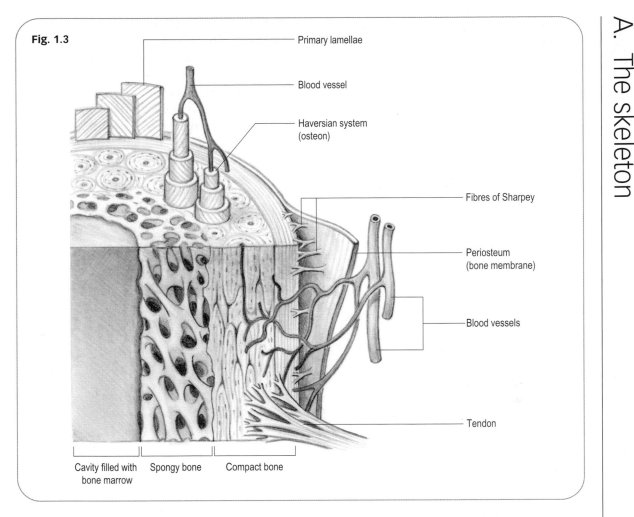

Fig. 1.3

Primary lamellae

Blood vessel

Haversian system (osteon)

Fibres of Sharpey

Periosteum (bone membrane)

Blood vessels

Tendon

Cavity filled with bone marrow   Spongy bone   Compact bone

so-called Haversian canal through which a small blood vessel runs. This blood vessel supplies the many layers with nourishment. Such a system is called a Haversian system, or osteon.

The outer layers of the bone form a system of longitudinal lamellae (layers). The tough collagenous fibres run in different directions in each layer, which considerably enhances the strength of the bone. The bone within the lamellae is made up of osteons. Farthest in towards the medullary cavity, the compact bone becomes so-called spongy tissue. In the compact and spongy tissues are reinforcing bars or braces that give the bone its great strength.

Figure 1.4 shows how these bars are aligned in the neck of the femur (femoral neck) in order to withstand the considerable stress to which this part of the bone is subjected. In the spongy bone and in the bone cavity you will find bone marrow,

which consists of immature cells that will develop into all sorts of blood cells.

The muscle tendons and ligaments are attached to the bone by collagenous fibres growing through the periosteum (bone membrane) and into the compact-bone tissue. When subjected to severe stress a tendon may hold, but its attachment to the bone may give way. A piece of the bone may thus be torn off or avulsed.

Where the muscle's tendon of attachment passes through the periosteum – which is rich in nerve and blood cells – an unfavourable stress can irritate the membrane and lead to periostitis (inflammation of the periosteum) (see p. 77).

In the deeper layer of the periosteum there are many bone-forming cells (osteoblasts), which are responsible for the repair of broken bones (fractures). The bone is supplied with

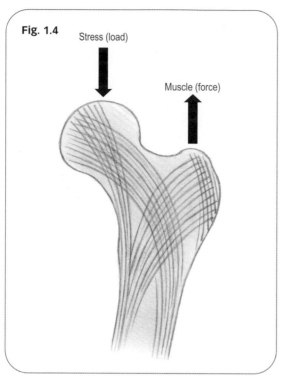

Fig. 1.4

Stress (load)

Muscle (force)

Attachments (membranes, ligaments, discs)

Between the tibia (shin bone) and the fibula (calf bone) there is a uniting membrane (interosseous membrane) comprised of collagenous fibrous tissues. It has two functions: (1) it serves as an origin for many of the muscles of the lower leg (see p. 76), and (2) it transmits stress from the tibia to the fibula. For example, when landing from a jump, force is exerted on the talus (ankle bone) and up through the tibia, but is then transmitted via the interosseus membrane to the fibula. (The tibia is thus relieved of some stress) (Figure 1.5).

The tibia and fibula are also united by two strong bands of fibrous tissue at the ankle (inferior

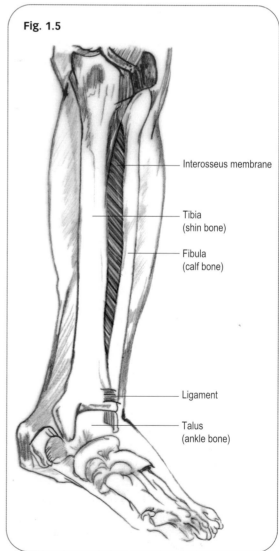

Fig. 1.5

Interosseus membrane

Tibia (shin bone)

Fibula (calf bone)

Ligament

Talus (ankle bone)

nutrients by the vast number of blood vessels that penetrate the compact tissue via the periosteum. The vessels then ramify and reach the different parts of the bone through the Haversian canals. The ability of the bone to repair itself is directly dependent upon the adequacy of the blood supply to the injured area. For example, when a metacarpal (one of the bones of the hand) is injured it often takes a long time to heal as there are few blood vessels in the area and, moreover, those that do exist are usually injured in the fracture.

Scientific investigation has revealed that the number of capillaries supplying muscles and bone increases if the muscles and bones are regularly subjected to stress (by training). This could explain the observation that injuries sustained by well-trained people heal much faster than those sustained by untrained people.

B. Joints

The different parts of the skeleton are connected either by attachments, such as membranes, or by joints.

tibiofibular joint). Such powerful, clearly distinguishable bands are called ligaments.

If the foot is violently pressed up against the lower leg (extension or dorsiflexion), the talus may wedge in between the fibula and tibia with such force that the anterior of the two ligaments may tear (rupture). The lower part of the interosseous membrane may also rupture.

Other examples of clearly distinguishable free ligaments are the crossed, or cruciate, ligaments that cross each other inside the knee joint as shown in Figure 1.6. Here the knee, without a patella (kneecap), is viewed from the front.

Another type of ligament provides reinforcement in the capsule that encloses a joint. This ligament is responsible for blocking those movements whose deviations are too great. It also restricts movements in certain directions.

The strongest of all the ligaments in the body (iliofemoral ligament) (Figure 1.7) is a thickened band of fibres situated on the frontal aspect of the hip capsule. It restricts excessive backward swings of the legs. The strength of a ligament or tendon can be 5000–10 000 N/cm^2

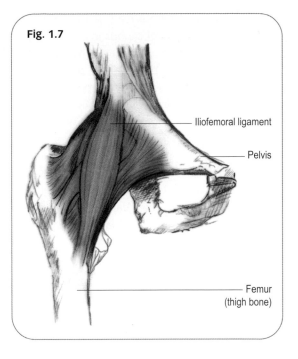

Fig. 1.7

Iliofemoral ligament

Pelvis

Femur
(thigh bone)

of cross-section. The iliofemoral ligament in an adult person can withstand a stress of 3000 N.

Another type of attachment can be found between the vertebrae of the spinal column. It is composed not only of collagenous fibres, but also of cartilage cells; and in its centre is a soft nucleus (Figure 1.8). The overall structure is called an intervertebral disc; it is an example of

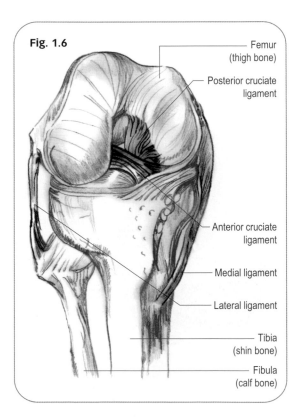

Fig. 1.6

Femur
(thigh bone)

Posterior cruciate
ligament

Anterior cruciate
ligament

Medial ligament

Lateral ligament

Tibia
(shin bone)

Fibula
(calf bone)

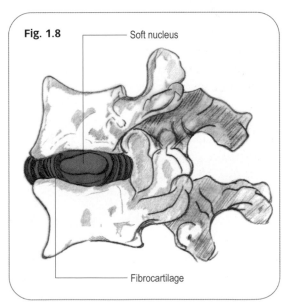

Fig. 1.8

Soft nucleus

Fibrocartilage

a secondary cartilaginous joint. A further example of this type of cartilaginous joint is the symphysis pubis (pubic symphysis) (Figure 1.9) connecting the pubic bones of the pelvis.

Additional examples of joint types are that of the epiphyseal cartilage (a primary cartilaginous joint) (see p. 2), and the fibrous joint between the flat bones of the skull (suture) (Figure 1.10).

Joints (synovial joints)

The surfaces of the bones of a synovial joint are always enclosed in a joint capsule and they are always covered with articular cartilage. The outer layer of the capsule is formed by collagen fibres, which are highly resistant to force. The powerful reinforcements of the capsule wall are called ligaments (see Figure 1.7). They receive their names according to their position or according to the bones they connect.

In the inner layer of the capsule there are cells that produce a fluid containing albumin. This fluid acts as a lubricant and provides the cartilage cells with nutrients. It is called synovial fluid and the membrane that lines the capsule is called the synovial membrane. The inner and outer layers are separated by a thin layer of fat (Figure 1.11).

The thickness of the cartilage of a joint depends on the stress to which it is normally subjected. The cartilage is able to absorb certain substances from the synovial fluid and swell temporarily. If we were to measure the size of the articular cartilage after a period of warming up, we would find that it had thickened. The thickening is only temporary, lasting for 10–30 minutes after the activity has ceased. Prolonged training causes the cartilage to thicken by the formation of additional cartilage cells. However, severe or uneven stress can wear the cartilage down, resulting in seriously restricted movement at the joint.

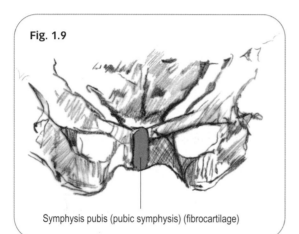

Fig. 1.9

Symphysis pubis (pubic symphysis) (fibrocartilage)

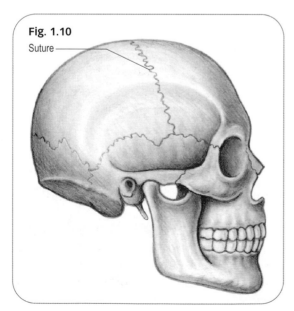

Fig. 1.10

Suture

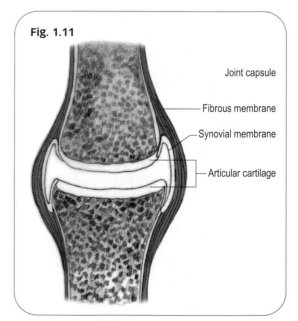

Fig. 1.11

Joint capsule

Fibrous membrane

Synovial membrane

Articular cartilage

Little sacs of synovial fluid (bursae) are found associated with certain joints; they are formed in the same way as the joint capsule.

The bursa's inner layer (synovial membrane) causes it to form a displacement cushion with very low friction.

The bursa's task is, above all, to prevent wear of the different structures that glide over each other. However, it also produces synovial fluid in those cases where it is connected with a joint.

The largest bursa of the body (the suprapatellar bursa) is situated between the femur (thigh bone) and the knee extensors (the quadriceps femoris or four-headed thigh muscle) (Figure 1.12). When the knee is subjected to severe stress, the bursa becomes sore. It reacts by producing extra quantities of synovial fluid. This leads to a swelling of the knee (water on the knee), which prevents further stress.

Bursae can be found in many different places in the body. For example, between muscles, between tendons and muscles, and between tendons and bone, i.e. wherever wear and tear is likely.

The bones that make up a joint generally fit together well. Usually one of the bones is convex (the head) and the other is concave (the socket or depression). If, however, the bones do not fit together well, the irregularities are evened out by extra layers of fibrocartilage. These inclusions are called menisci if they only partly subdivide a joint cavity. If the joint is completely partitioned into two separate parts, the layer of fibrocartilage is called a disc.

In sports injuries, references to menisci usually apply to those of the knee, although one can also find menisci between other bones of the body. For example, between the clavicle (collar bone) and the scapula (shoulder blade) (Figure 1.13).

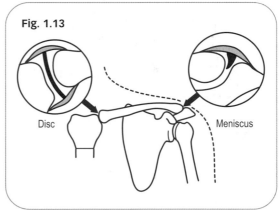

Fig. 1.13

Disc　　　　　　　　　　　　　　Meniscus

Different types of joints

The function of joints is usually described with the aid of mechanical models. However, there is not always a close resemblance between mechanical models and the actual joints of the human body. The diagrams below show different types of joints along with the parts of the body where they can be found. In addition, illustrations are given of the type of movement allowed by these joints.

Because the capsular ligament around a gliding joint (Figure 1.14) is almost always taut, the movements allowed at such joints are described as small but multidirectional (hence multiaxial).

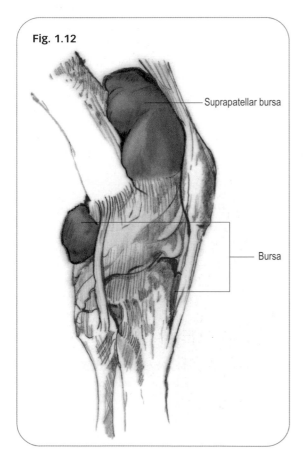

Fig. 1.12

Suprapatellar bursa

Bursa

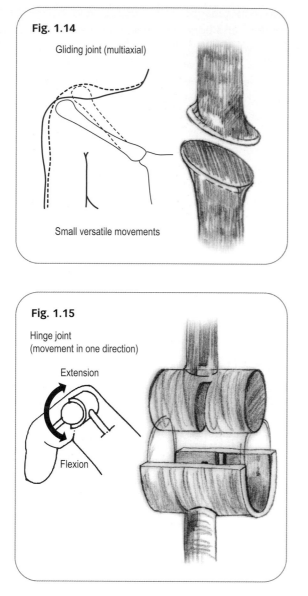

Fig. 1.14

Gliding joint (multiaxial)

Small versatile movements

Fig. 1.15

Hinge joint
(movement in one direction)

Extension

Flexion

Fig. 1.16

Pivot joint
(movement in one plane only)

Pronation

Supination

Fig. 1.17

Saddle joint
(movements round two axes)

Adduction
(movements towards
the midline of the body)

Flexion

Extension

Abduction
(movements away from
the midline of the body)

Many of the body's joints have designs that cannot be related to any of the models shown in Figures 1.14–1.19. Instead, a combination of two models or one of the models with some modification is used for descriptive purposes. For example, the knee joint is a combination of a hinge and a pivot joint (Figures 1.15–1.16 give examples of hinge and pivot). At that joint, flexion and extension are possible as well as inward and outward rotation of the lower leg, but the leg can only be rotated when the knee is bent. Figure 1.20 shows the maximum range of movement in the knee joint.

The third knuckle joints are modified ball and socket joints (Figure 1.19). The head of one bone and the socket of the other correspond almost exactly to the ball and socket model, but the capsular ligament prevents certain movements and there are no muscles for rotating the finger.

Of all the muscles that protect the joint from injury, those that directly surround it are the most important. A strong and supple musculature is always the best protection against joint injuries. Violent physical activity can lead to different kinds of muscle injuries. Muscles can be overstretched, partly ruptured or even completely

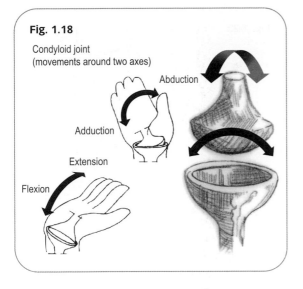

Fig. 1.18

Condyloid joint
(movements around two axes)

Abduction

Adduction

Extension

Flexion

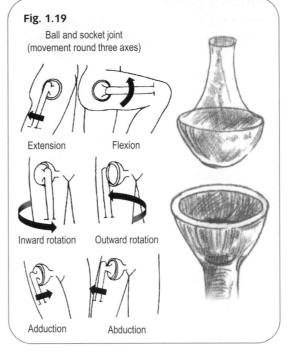

Fig. 1.19

Ball and socket joint
(movement round three axes)

Extension   Flexion

Inward rotation   Outward rotation

Adduction   Abduction

ruptured. When a ligament is stretched, it usually returns to its original length and function after some weeks of rest.

If the same ligament is repeatedly stretched, the result can be a slack, non-functional ligament. The joint then only fits loosely together, which can lead to serious injury. Such a ligament should be shortened by surgery. Ligaments that are completely torn should be sewn together. Partially torn ligaments can be operated on and sewn together, but if the torn parts are in contact they can heal if the affected area is kept still. In such cases the joint should be set in a cast. In recent years, it has been shown that even a completely torn Achilles tendon (heel tendon), heals if the ankle is set in such a position that the parts of the tendon lie against each other.

A ligament can be made slack and unstressed by taping. The aim of taping a joint is to prevent movements that can strain a weak or injured ligament. Taping in athletics is defensible after injury has been sustained or as part of an effort to prevent injury when it is known that the risk of injury is high (e.g. in vigorous football training, or other competitive situations). However, an athlete should avoid the habitual use of taping during training as this could lead to an injury of the skin. Moreover, the unloaded ligament becomes accustomed to external help after a while, and is thus weakened.

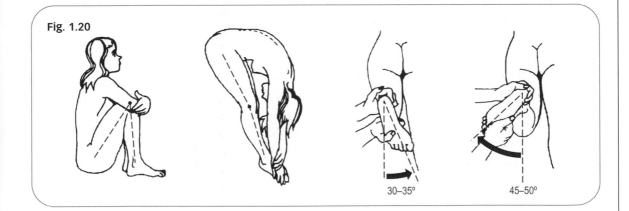

Fig. 1.20

30–35°   45–50°

Different planes

When describing movements you assume that the person is standing in the so-called anatomic starting position (Figure 1.21). You then systematize the movements imagining that these can take place in three planes through the body (Figure 1.21).

The plane going through the body from side to side is called the frontal plane. Outward movement of structures within the frontal plane is called abduction (Figure 1.22A).

When the movement involves returning to or going beyond the starting position, the movement is called adduction.

The front-to-back plane is the median plane. Movements in parallel with this plane are called flexion or extension. If you move from the starting position to the position shown in Figure 1.22B a flexion occurs in all joints involved in the movement (except within the toes). The muscles responsible for the movement are termed the flexors. To return to the starting position the antagonists of the flexors come into play.

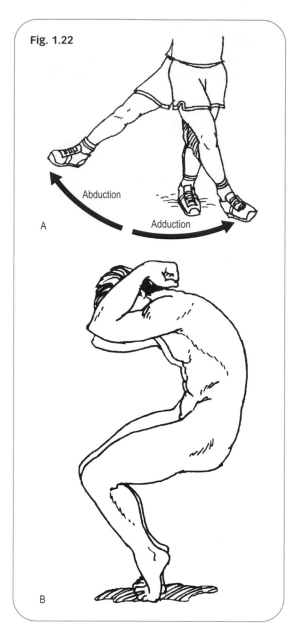

Fig. 1.22

Abduction

Adduction

A

B

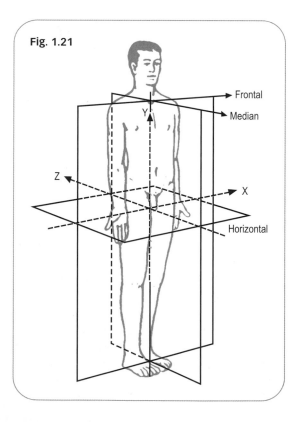

Fig. 1.21

Frontal

Median

Y

Z

X

Horizontal

They are called extensors and the movements that occur in the different joints are called extensions.

The third and last plane that is used to describe the body's ability to move is called the horizontal plane.

Movements in this plane (Figure 1.23) are called outward rotation or inward rotation. In the so-called anatomic starting position the hand and the lower arm should be rotated outwardly almost to a maximum.

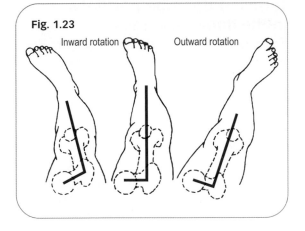

Fig. 1.23

Inward rotation   Outward rotation

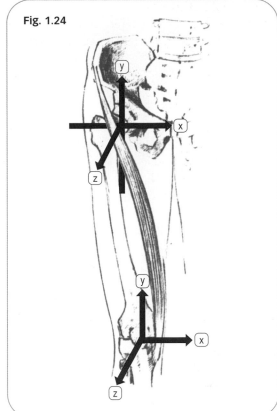

Fig. 1.24

Axes of motion

One way of describing joints is to say in how many of the planes, described above, movement can take place. This leads to joints being classified into three groups: one-axis joints allowing movement only in one plane, two-axes joints allowing movement in two of the planes, and three-axes joints allowing movement in all three planes. In Figure 1.24 the three different axes are marked as x-, y- and z-axes. Around the z-axis abduction and adduction take place. Around the x-axis flexion and extension take place. Around the y-axis outward and inward rotation take place. One example of a muscle with several functions in a joint, because its pulling force lies to the side of all the axes of movement involved, is the sartorius (tailor's muscle) (Figure 1.24). This muscle runs from the upper anterior (frontal) part of the pelvis, across the thigh down to the tibia (shin bone). To be able to understand the different functions one has to judge where the muscle lies in relation to the different axes. Looking at the z-axis, it can be seen that the muscle lies outside the axis. This indicates that the movement that the muscle produces is an abduction. Looking at the x-axis, it can be seen that the muscle passes in front of the axis, indicating that the muscle will produce a flexion in the joint. Around the y-axis there is an outward rotation depending on the pulling force lying outside and anterior to the axis. In the knee joint the muscle passes behind the x-axis and inside–posterior to the y-axis,

which means it produces flexion and inward rotation. The final position of the leg after the muscle has contracted and all five movements have taken place resembles the way tailors used to sit when they worked. The name of the muscle is therefore the tailor's muscle, which is a direct translation from the Latin *musculus sartorius*.

Because the sartorius is a long thin muscle, it is easy to see how (and where) it traverses the joints. This is illustrated in Figure 1.24.

The deltoideus (deltoid muscle) (Figure 1.25) has a large area of origin, such that some parts of the muscle pass in front of the x-axis and some parts pass behind the axis. In other words the muscle can produce both a flexion and an extension; this is possible because muscles have the ability to contract in certain parts while other parts rest. This is because muscle cells are controlled by nerve cells, located in the spinal marrow, each of which controls a number of muscle cells. Such a nerve cell, along with the muscle

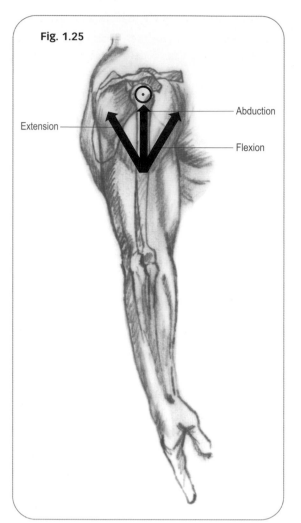

Fig. 1.25

Extension

Abduction

Flexion

Terms to describe positions in the body (Figure 1.26)

To be able to describe where in the body a certain muscle is placed, where a bone is situated in relation to another structure etc., sets of paired antithetical terms are used. These terms are often used in names of muscles, tendons, ligaments and bones.

Anterior/posterior are terms used to describe a structure situated forward/backward in the body. Musculus pectoralis major (the greater chest muscle) is placed anteriorly and the scapula (shoulder blade), posteriorly.

Superior/inferior are terms that are used to indicate positions upward/downward in the body (Figure 1.26). The hip bone as seen from the right-hand side in Figure 3.2, p. 52 shows four visible projections or spines, all of which are origins for the attachment of muscles or ligaments, and each having the name spina iliaca (iliac spine). Their anatomic positions are then described using the two sets of terms given above. One spine (which is the origin for musculus sartorius (tailor's muscle)) is consequently called spina iliaca anterior superior. The origin for musculus rectus femoris (straight thigh muscle) is spina iliaca anterior inferior.

cells that it innervates, is called a motor unit. A motor unit in the deltoideus can be placed so that it only contributes to one movement, for example a flexion, even if the entire muscle can bring about two or three different types of motion. When other motor units in the muscle operate there can be an extension. If a certain combination of units are active, flexion and extension block each other; as a result there will only be an abduction. Due to the way in which motor units are distributed, many muscles have the ability to perform several different functions. These different functions are dependent on where the mean force lies in relation to the different axes of movement.

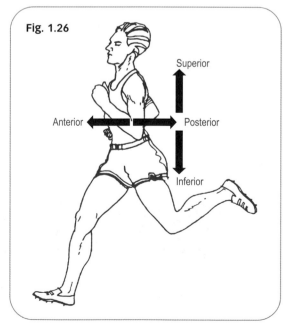

Fig. 1.26

Superior

Anterior

Posterior

Inferior

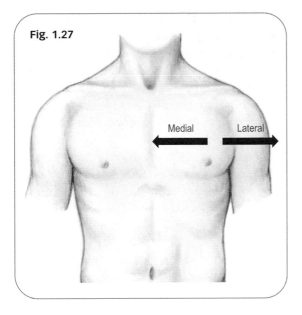

Fig. 1.27

Medial ← → Lateral

Lateral/medial are terms that describe something placed far away/close to the midline (Figure 1.27) of the body. In the knee, for example, there are two menisci. The one that is placed in the inside of the knee is called the meniscus medialis (internal meniscus) in contrast to the meniscus lateralis (external meniscus). We also refer to the medial (internal) and lateral (external) collateral ligaments of a joint; these give stability to the joint. In the knee the meniscus medialis grows together with the medial collateral ligament, which is part of the reason why 80% of all the injuries in the menisci affect the meniscus medialis. The lateral meniscus is placed in a more spacious position and may glide away easily if extreme and harmful movements of the knee joint take place (Figure 3.32, p. 62).

There are a few additional pairs of terms that describe positions in the body (e.g. caudal, abdominal, proximal, distal, etc.), but those most frequently used are mentioned above.

C. Muscles

There are three different types of muscles in the body: smooth muscle, cardiac muscle and skeletal muscle. This book will only deal with the last of these, which is also called striated, or striped, muscle.

Skeletal muscle is surrounded by a layer of connective tissue. The connective tissue is built up in the same way as the outer layer of a joint capsule (see p. 6). Its task is to provide a surface against which the surrounding muscles can glide, and it gives a muscle its form.

The layer of connective tissue is called the muscle's fascia, or epimysium. The connective tissue consists mainly of collagen fibres. Looking at a section of a muscle with the naked eye, we see that it is made up of small cell bundles (fasciculi). Each of the fasciculi is surrounded by a thin layer of connective tissue whose Latin name is perimysium. In the perimysium – which is made up of both collagenous and elastic fibres – the nerve and blood vessels branch off before finally reaching the actual muscle cells. Under the microscope we can see that each fasciculus consists of a number of muscle cells. Each muscle cell is surrounded by a very thin layer of connective tissue, which is called endomysium (endo = internal; mys = muscle).

The muscle cell is also called a muscle fibre; thus a muscle fibre consists of a single cell. The

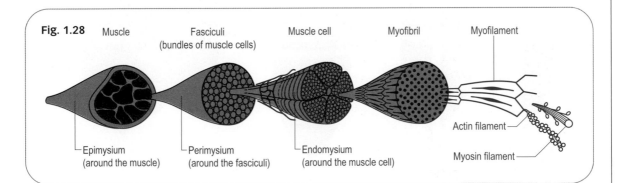

Fig. 1.28

Muscle

Fasciculi (bundles of muscle cells)

Muscle cell

Myofibril

Myofilament

Actin filament

Myosin filament

Epimysium (around the muscle)

Perimysium (around the fasciculi)

Endomysium (around the muscle cell)

structure and function of muscle cells is described very thoroughly in the majority of books on physiology. The following account is therefore brief.

When examined under the microscope, the muscle cell is seen to be composed of small structures called muscle fibrils or myofibrils. The fibrils lie in parallel and give the muscle cell a striated appearance. This is because the fibrils are made up of smaller components – myofilaments – which are regularly aligned.

Myofilaments are chains of protein molecules (Figure 1.28). The striated appearance is due to the presence of two types of myofilament,

namely, actin (which is thinner than myosin and colours more lightly with the stains used in microscopy) and myosin (which is thicker than actin and is responsible for the darker-staining bands).

When the muscle contracts, the actin filaments move longitudinally between the myosin filaments. As a consequence, the myofibrils shorten and thicken.

The connective tissue surrounding the muscle, the epimysium, extends and is continuous with the muscle's tendon. The muscles of the body have very different shapes. Figure 1.29 shows the most common variations.

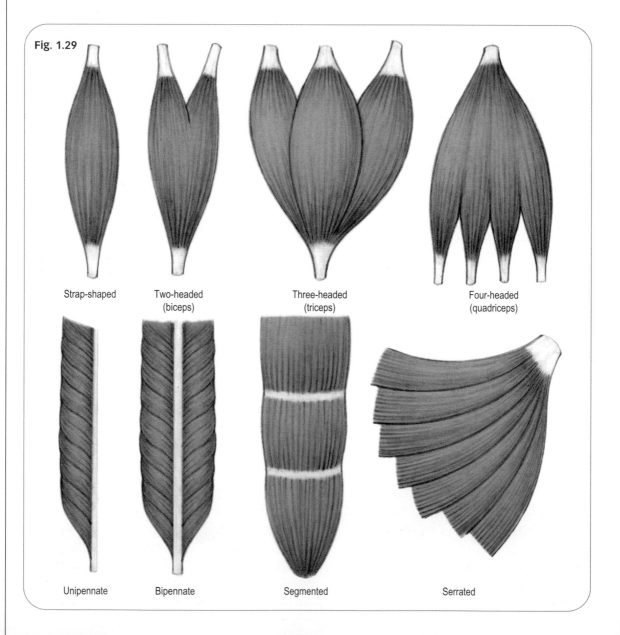

Fig. 1.29

Strap-shaped

Two-headed (biceps)

Three-headed (triceps)

Four-headed (quadriceps)

Unipennate

Bipennate

Segmented

Serrated

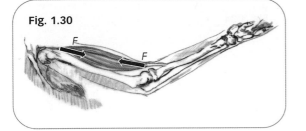

Fig. 1.30

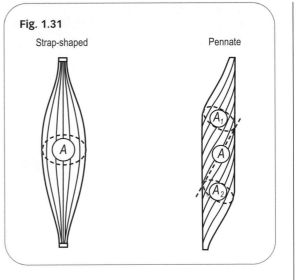

Fig. 1.31

Strap-shaped   Pennate

When a muscle contracts, it produces a force (F) (Figure 1.30) that affects the origin and insertion of the muscle equally, but in opposite directions.

A muscle can develop a maximal force of about 50 N/cm² of the muscle's cross-section. The cross-section referred to here is physiological, and it is defined in the following way: if the cells of a muscle run longitudinally in a muscle that has a strap-shaped appearance as in Figure 1.31, the geometrical cross-section of the muscle (A) will provide a measurement of how many actin and myosin filaments are contained in the muscle. If the area is 6 cm², the maximal force of contraction will be $6 \times 50 = 300$ N. However, if the muscle cells run diagonally in relation to the muscle's longitudinal direction, as shown in the pennate muscle in Figure 1.31, then the areas A_1 and A_2 must be measured in order to arrive at the total number of actin and myosin filaments contained in the muscle.

$A_1 + A_2$ gives the muscle's physiological cross-section. If $A_1 = 8$ cm² and $A_2 = 4$ cm², the muscle's physiological cross-section will be 12 cm². The muscle's maximal strength is $12 \times 50 = 600$ N. This muscle is thus considerably stronger than the strap-shaped muscle, even if both muscles have equal mass. A single muscle cell can shorten its length by about 50%. (For a whole muscle the figure is about 30%.) (Figure 1.32). The strap-shaped muscle can therefore be shortened over a greater distance than the pennate muscle.

The strap-shaped muscle is found in places where it is necessary to execute large ranges of movement quickly. Pennate-shaped muscles, on the other hand, can be found where movements over a small range but of great strength are required.

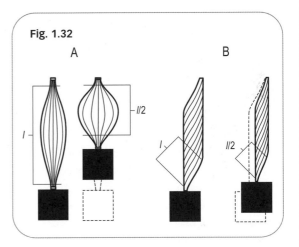

Fig. 1.32

A   B

The alignment of force of a muscle is dependent on the physiological cross-section. The ability to contract depends on the length of the fleshy part measured in the direction of alignment of the cells. In order to assess the effect of a muscle we must also know where it is attached in relation to the joint.

Figure 1.33A shows that if a muscle is attached 4 cm from the joint axis, its contraction force must be 700 N if it is to support a weight of 7 kg located 40 cm from the joint ($700 \times 4 = 70 \times 40$). If, instead, the same muscle were attached 5 cm from the joint, then its force need only be 560 N ($560 \times 5 = 70 \times 40$) (Figure 1.33B). The ability of a muscle to lift a heavy object is thus dependent on two factors: its

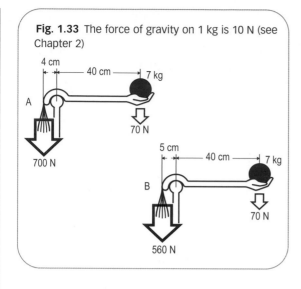

Fig. 1.33 The force of gravity on 1 kg is 10 N (see Chapter 2)

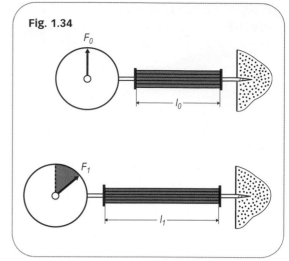

Fig. 1.34

physiological cross-section and its position in relation to the joint. A muscle's strength is more adequately described when we know its ability to develop the moment of force (M), as well as its force of contraction. (The concept 'moment of force' is described in Chapter 2.)

Relationship between developed force and length for a muscle

A piece of a muscle cut out to examine how much force the muscle can produce shows that the thicker the cell bunch is, the more force the muscle piece can produce. The contraction force depends mainly on the number of muscle cells taking part in the contraction, but it also depends upon the distance between origin and insertion when the muscle receives its contraction impulse. It is the brain cells that send the electric signal that initiates the contraction of a muscle in the body. In the laboratory two electrodes are used to produce the signal. If we suppose that we have cut out a part of a muscle with the length of l_0 and fastened it between two steady plates, where one plate is working as a force meter, we will be able to examine how much force can be generated, depending on the distance between origin and insertion.

What generates the force in general is the ability of the actin filaments of the muscle fibre to 'climb' along the myosin filaments via the swinging-movements of the so-called cross-bridges (Figure 1.35). The 'climbing' can only occur for a certain distance, after which the actin from one end meets the actin from the other end. The repeating units to which this description applies are called sarcomeres. A sarcomere is the part between two transverse partitions (Z-bands) (Figure 1.35).

In our imagined laboratory test this fact is demonstrated since the muscle cannot contract enough to produce any force at all when the distance between the attachment plates is less than 50% of l_0. When the distance is: (A) 75%,

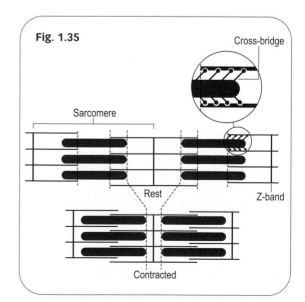

Fig. 1.35

(B) 100%, or (C) 120% of l_0 (Figure 1.36) the contraction force increases according to the graph in the bottom of the figure.

The explanation of the graph in Figure 1.37 is as follows.

If the muscle is extended (see l_1 in Figure 1.34) or in other words stretched by some external force (by the muscles' antagonists (counteracting muscles) or by a movement causing origin and insertion to become separated by more than l_0), its ability to contract will be dependent in part on the tendency of its elastic parts to return to the original position (the rubber-band effect) and in part on its ability to contract by way of its actin filaments climbing over the myosin filaments. The elasticity contribution to the total ability to contract follows the black dotted line in the upper graph of Figure 1.37.

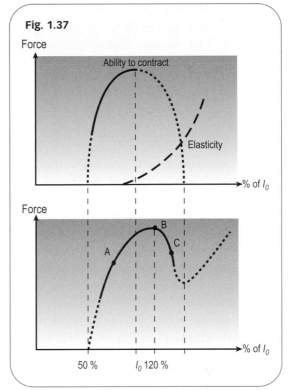

Fig. 1.37

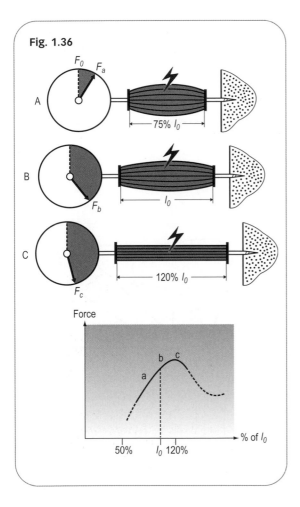

Fig. 1.36

The red curve in the upper part of Figure 1.37 illustrates the force component that depends on the active ability of actin–myosin interactions to cause contraction. The actual contraction force can be deduced by combining the two contributions to give the bottom curve. Since the elasticity curve rises more steeply than the actin–myosin curve decreases (in the area of 120% of l_0), the contraction curve will increase if the muscle is pulled apart, and with electric stimuli the muscle is forced to contract in a static way between the two attachment plates. The total contraction force will be at its maximum when the distance between origin and insertion is 20% longer than in the resting position (l_0). The laboratory test shows that when the muscle preparation is extended to an extreme, only the elasticity force remains. In this case, the ability of the actin filaments to climb over the myosin filaments is lost. In reality, ligaments or the construction of the skeleton usually prevent excessively large movements; most of the muscles operate within the area that is shown by the solid line in the graph in Figure 1.36.

You can do a small unscientific test of what is described above by testing the grip strength in one hand. The muscles that originate in the area around the inner part of the elbow flex the wrist but also cause the fingers to grip. Test your strength in your right hand by gripping around your left thumb as hard as you can (Figure 1.38).

If you bend the wrist of the hand with which you are gripping, then in positions (A), (B) or (C) in Figure 1.38, you will basically be at points (A), (B) or (C) in Figure 1.37. You will develop the most power at (B), because the length between the origin and the insertion of the muscle is optimal. You then hold a grip so you only need to use a low percentage of your strength but there is the possibility to squeeze with maximum force if needed.

Another test could be to sit behind a person who is withdrawing his legs as in the position shown in Figure 1.39. You will notice that the force is small in (A), greater in (B) and a little smaller again in (C). This test is also a little unscientific since the muscle's lever to the joint is not the same in all three positions. However, one gets an idea of how the force varies in different positions and a feeling of the muscles having a strength profile. Strength profile refers to muscle strength in different parts of the range of motion.

Further information about this will be given in Chapter 2.

Another example of a muscle's ability to generate force can be indicated in the position shown in Figure 1.40.

When you touch the Achilles tendon (heel tendon) you will notice that it is difficult to generate any tension because the origin and the insertion for the gastrocnemius (twin calf muscle) are too close to each other. If you change the angle in the knee or ankle joint it will become easier to contract the muscle.

In a standing jump from a knees bent start the gastrocnemius does not contract and lift the heel from the ground until the knee extension is almost completely finished. The straighter the knee the longer is the gastrocnemius, everything depending on the distance between origin and insertion according to the above discussion.

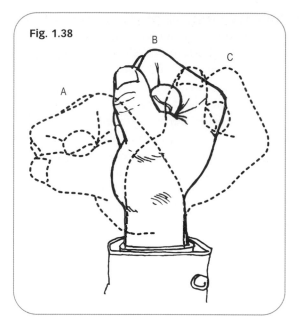

Fig. 1.38

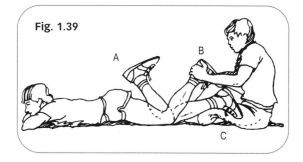

Fig. 1.39

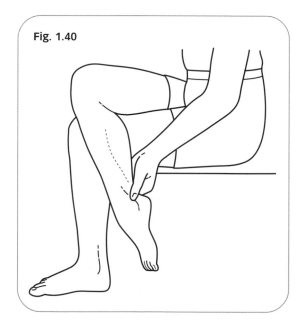

Fig. 1.40

Different types of muscular work

When observing the way muscles work, it is usual to distinguish between dynamic and static work.

Dynamic work means that the origin and insertion of a muscle are forcefully affected by changes in muscle length. If the muscular force causes the origin and insertion to move towards each other, we say that the muscle works concentrically (the muscle is shortened, contracted). If the muscle force is exerted while the origin and insertion are receding from each other (i.e. the muscle tries to halt a movement in a joint), the muscle is said to work eccentrically (although the muscle tries to shorten, it is actually lengthened by external forces).

When a muscle contracts without any movement taking place in the joint, it is said that the muscle acts statically (or isometrically). Figures 1.41 and 1.42 show how the flexors and the extensors in the elbow joint work.

Figure 1.43 shows a training exercise that provides concentric work for the lumbar muscles (the movement takes place mainly at the small of the back), and static effort for the neck and chest muscles. During descent, the lumbar muscles work eccentrically in an effort to halt the movement. (For the back muscles, see p. 94.)

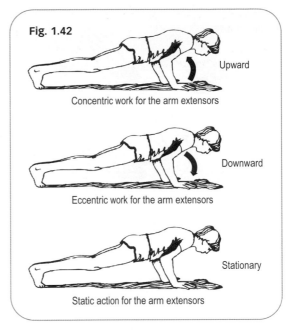

Fig. 1.42

Upward

Concentric work for the arm extensors

Downward

Eccentric work for the arm extensors

Stationary

Static action for the arm extensors

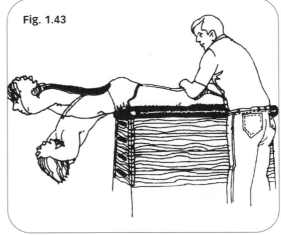

Fig. 1.43

Figure 1.44 shows what happens when a person sits up from a lying position.

1–2. Concentric work primarily for the rectus abdominis (straight abdominal muscle) (p. 98).

2–3. Static action for the abdominal muscles, concentric for the hip flexors (p. 58).

3–4. Almost no work for the abdominal muscles. Concentric work for the hip flexors.

4. Static action for the back extensors.

It is easier to analyse the exercises that are used in competitive sports, strength training,

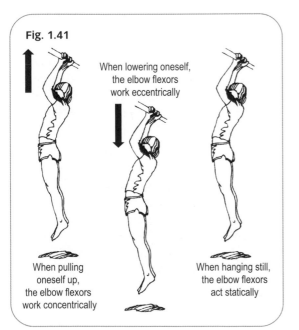

Fig. 1.41

When lowering oneself, the elbow flexors work eccentrically

When pulling oneself up, the elbow flexors work concentrically

When hanging still, the elbow flexors act statically

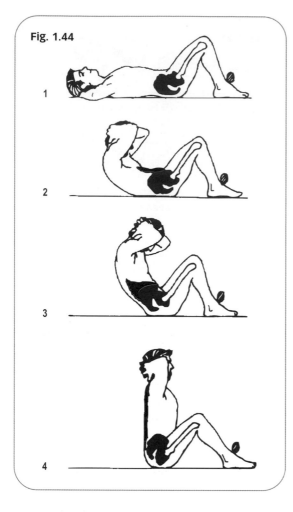

Fig. 1.44

1

2

3

4

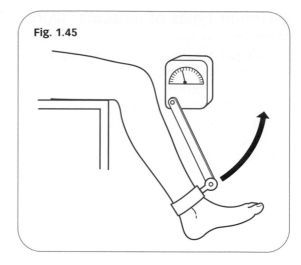

Fig. 1.45

flexibility training, etc., when we know the origin and insertion of muscles. Physiological studies have shown that if a muscle is exercised concentrically, its ability to work statically and eccentrically is not appreciably increased. We can assume that the reason for this lies in the fact that the muscle's ability to work is dependent partly on its mass and partly on its supply of nerve impulses. Both these functions must operate for the muscle to be effective. A good athlete or trainer ought to be capable of analysing the particular branch of athletics and designing exercises to meet the demands of the movements involved.

Relationship between developed force and contraction speed for a muscle

This relationship has mainly been mapped with the help of a so-called isokinetic dynamometer.

The tested person (Tp) presses against an arm of the chair, while seated; this arm turns round an axis lying parallel to that of the knee joint (Figure 1.45).

There is a meter on the arm of the chair showing the force with which the knee extensor muscle, the quadriceps femoris (four-headed thigh muscle), contracts. With this apparatus you can, for example, find out the Tp's maximal isometric force for a 90° angle in the knee joint. The chair is constructed so that an engine can drive the arm at different speeds. You can, for example, set the arm's movement at 60°/s. You ask the Tp to press as much as possible while the arm is moving at the pre-set speed. If you read off the force when the lower leg is positioned such that the angle in the knee is 90° you will be able to compare the isometric force generated with the force when the angle speed is 60°/s. Through varying the speed from 0 to 720°/s you will see how the concentric force depends on the speed of rotation in the joint. The apparatus can also be turned in the opposite direction with the Tp attempting to brake the movement; in this case the muscles work eccentrically. Figure 1.46 gives a graphic representation of the above.

Animal testing has given results indicating that the braking power can exceed the isometric maximum by up to 80%. In laboratory tests on human beings the curve for eccentric work depends a great deal on motivation and fear of getting hurt etc. The results are normally values

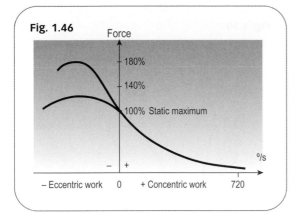

Fig. 1.46

Force

180%

140%

100% Static maximum

°/s

− +

− Eccentric work   0   + Concentric work   720

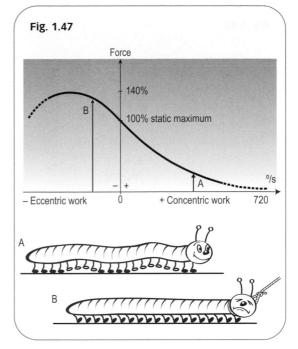

Fig. 1.47

Force

140%

B

100% static maximum

− +   A   °/s

− Eccentric work   0   + Concentric work   720

A

B

just over the isometric maximum. In an emergency situation, values higher than those found in the laboratory are expected.

To simplify matters we could liken the situation to the movements of a caterpillar (see Figure 1.47(A)). Suppose that a caterpillar is 'walking' slowly straight ahead. Most of its feet can be on the ground at the same time and help build up force. The feet will in this context represent the connections (bridges) between actin and myosin filaments. At a higher speed there are fewer feet in contact with the ground and consequently the force will be less. At very high speeds, the legs' backward movement will be too slow to contribute any more force to the movement. The maximum speed has been reached.

With the eccentric work (B), you can figuratively imagine that the caterpillar has all its feet on the ground and tries to hold back with all its power. In reality, the body is likely to have a better ability to mobilize a greater number of muscle units at braking since this is a movement that causes injuries if there is insufficient time for the braking movement to be performed efficiently.

Suppose that you are doing a standing jump as high as you can. The muscles work concentrically with powers that are represented by arrow A in Figure 1.47. We suppose the height of the jump to be about 50 cm. On landing, the same muscles are used as when you jump up, but now these are working eccentrically (B). This gives you greater force and can therefore brake the movement before you sink down too far and hurt, for example, your knees.

One can also speculate that movements can be done more efficiently because of the unique relationship between eccentric and concentric force. Suppose that you are going to kick as fast as possible (Figure 1.48). First, the lower leg accelerates with help from the quadriceps femoris. Then the leg has to brake before it reaches the final position, otherwise the knee would get injured by overstretching. The muscles that brake are placed on the back side of the knee (hamstrings) and work eccentrically in the braking movement. If these muscles were weaker than the quadriceps femoris, the accelerating phase would have to be interrupted at an early stage so that the braking could be carried out in time. This would result in a lower speed for the lower leg before interruption of the acceleration. If the braking muscles were very strong they could wait until very late in the movement before starting to interrupt it in order to protect the joint. This would afford the possibility of a longer acceleration phase for the quadriceps femoris and, as a result, a higher maximal speed in the movement.

When we want to obtain the maximal speed in a movement, a good technique involves working the muscles under the most favourable conditions possible.

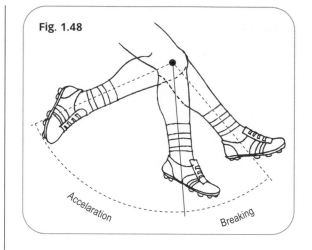

Fig. 1.48

Accelaration

Breaking

The hip muscle that is engaged when the leg is pushed forcefully backwards (Figure 1.49) is the gluteus maximus (large buttock muscle).

When a person walks on level ground they do not need to push off from the ground with high force, but if they encounter a steep ascent, they automatically bend forwards. Thus, the gluteus maximus is lengthened so that the force developed is greater (120% as shown above).

Think about what a person does to increase their speed when skating, running or cycling.

In order to give a football a mighty kick (Figure 1.50), for example, the thigh must start from a position well behind the hip because an important knee extensor muscle (p. 64) passes over the hip joint. If the muscle is required to develop much force, then the distance between its origin and insertion must be greater than l_0.

For efficient throwing (Figure 1.51), it is necessary to lengthen an important group of muscles, represented in Figure 1.51 by the chest

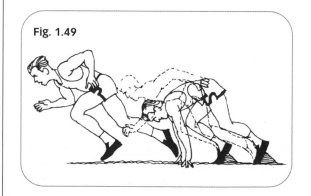

Fig. 1.49

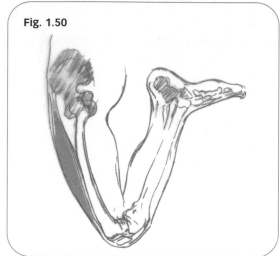

Fig. 1.50

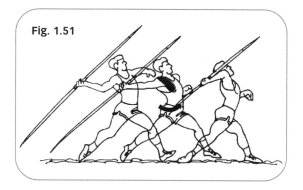

Fig. 1.51

muscle (p. 115). This group is stretched in relation to the arm when the trunk rotates fully in the opposite direction. At the same time, the chest is expanded by inhaling deeply.

D. Muscles–nervous system

The muscle's protective reflexes

There are two types of nerve cell that protect a muscle against unnecessary injuries: muscle spindles and tendon spindles.

Muscle spindles

The muscle spindles are connected in parallel to different muscle cells throughout the muscle. The muscle spindles passively follow the movements of their adjacent muscle cells.

When the muscle cells stretch, so do the muscle spindles. If the muscle stretches so much as to run the risk of being ruptured, the muscle spindle (Figure 1.52) responds by sending a signal to the muscle to contract. This keeps the muscle from being injured. This protective mechanism is called the stretch reflex.

When a doctor taps the ligament directly below the kneecap (ligamentum patellae) with a rubber mallet, the muscle cells in the knee-extensor muscles, the quadriceps femoris (four-headed thigh muscle), stretch (see p. 63). The muscle's reaction to this unexpected stretching is to protect itself by contracting – i.e. the knee jerks a little. The period of delay between the tap with the mallet and the kick is an indication of the time it takes the nerve impulse to travel from the muscle spindle to the spinal cord of the central nervous system (CNS) and back again to the muscle cells.

The centre of gravity (CG) of an adult's head lies above and in front of the joint that is anterior to the upper cervical vertebra (i.e. the uppermost vertebra of the neck) (Figure 1.53). The head is held upright – despite its natural tendency to tilt forward – by the tension maintained by the muscles of the neck. When a person falls asleep in a sitting position, the muscles of the neck relax, and the head falls forwards. The muscle

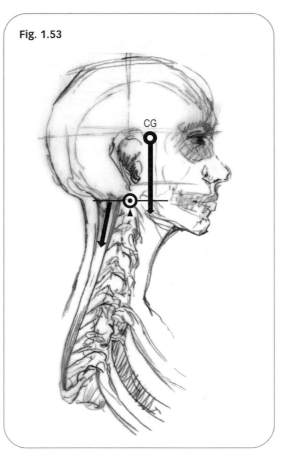

Fig. 1.53

CG

spindles stretch unexpectedly, which causes the head to jerk up. This protective mechanism has probably saved the lives of many a tired motorist and kept many a bored listener awake.

The protective mechanism of the muscle spindle responds when the muscle spindle is stretched unexpectedly, but it also permits voluntary stretches which are not too sudden. The head may be allowed to fall forward–downward without the reflex being evoked. It has been shown that if a muscle first contracts and then stretches slowly, it can be made to extend a little further. These principles should be carefully adhered to when training flexibility and movement. They are described in more detail on page 31.

In Figure 1.54 the spiral nerve endings that form the muscle spindle can be seen. Signals from these endings are sent to the spinal cord, which receives all the information coming from the environment. These signals are called afferent signals. The signals give continuous information about

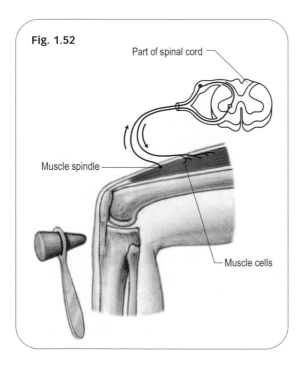

Fig. 1.52

Part of spinal cord

Muscle spindle

Muscle cells

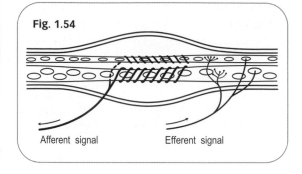

Fig. 1.54

Afferent signal   Efferent signal

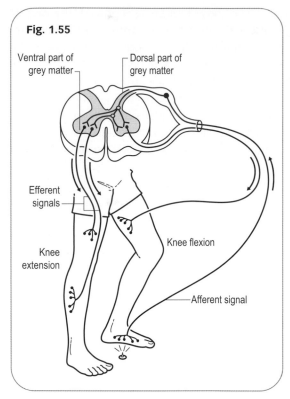

Fig. 1.55

Ventral part of grey matter   Dorsal part of grey matter

Efferent signals

Knee extension

Knee flexion

Afferent signal

position and length and thereby also the speed at which the muscle spindle moves. The movement of the muscle spindle is identical with the movement of the muscle since the spindle is connected (parallel) with the surrounding muscle cells. If the movement towards an outer position is too fast, activating signals will be sent out from the anterior part of the spinal cord and a reflex action will brake the movement. The afferent signals also give information if muscle force is too strong or too weak for its task, and in that case signals from the spinal cord adjust the power through disconnecting or connecting a number of motor units. The signals sent to the muscle cells from the spinal cord are called efferent signals and they all originate from the anterior part of the spinal cord. Some moving patterns are hereditary and are programmed in the nervous system; they are usually called reflexes. This means some reactions are subconscious (they occur without the person being aware of the reason for them).

If, for example, you step on a sharp object there will be an automatic movement involving the arms and the upper body so that the weight can be shifted on to the other foot, and the foot that hurts can be taken away (Figure 1.55). All this happens before the signals have reached the brain, where they are converted to pain. If pain had initiated the required actions to take the foot away, the movement would have taken more time and the injury would have been more serious.

When learning a new movement, corrections slowly take place and they are made consciously; in other words the brain receives the information that it processes before actions are made to correct possible faults. This takes time. The more

often a movement is repeated the fewer corrections have to be made by the motor cells in the brain and eventually it will take place like a reflex 'via the spinal cord'. Some researchers say that it takes some 10 000 repetitions before a movement becomes automatic. The part of the brain that sends out signals to the muscles of the body is called the centre for motor activity. The cells involved are concentrated in an area around the frontal and central lobes.

Figure 1.56 illustrates the relative number of cells that are used to control different body parts. As you can see, the muscles of the thumb are activated by a lot of nerve cells. The ability to grip with the thumb may be one of the reasons why the human being has developed into such a technical creature.

Tendon organs

Placed between the muscle cells and the tendon tissue are the tendon organs. A tendon organ is also called a Golgi organ (Figure 1.57).

In contrast to the muscle spindles the tendon organs give an inhibiting signal, in other words a

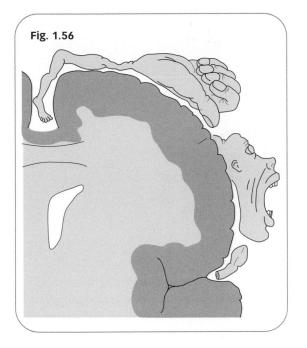

Fig. 1.56

muscle spindle are in the majority the muscle will be contracted. If the negative signals from the tendon organs, and thereby from the interneuron, are in the majority the contraction will be stopped.

Figures 1.58 and 1.59 illustrate two situations in which reflexes will give different results and also shows how the different sensory organs control the muscle. Imagine that you move your arm backwards quickly towards the outer position to do a maximal throw. If the arm has moved backwards too far on with too much speed towards an outer position, and there is a risk of a rupture, the muscle spindles will send a warning signal and the muscle will contract; the arm will then brake and turn back before it reaches the critical position.

Figure 1.59 illustrates the leg of a badminton player who is taking a step backwards to reach a shuttle cock at the same time as making a hard smash. His whole body weight is on its way backwards and downwards; his muscle (the triceps surae or three-headed calf muscle) is contracted to a maximum so that his heel will not sink down to the floor; instead he will move

signal that prevents the muscle from contracting. This occurs when a so-called interneuron receives the signal from the muscle spindle. This 'in-between cell' sends a negative signal to the motor nerve. If the positive signals from the

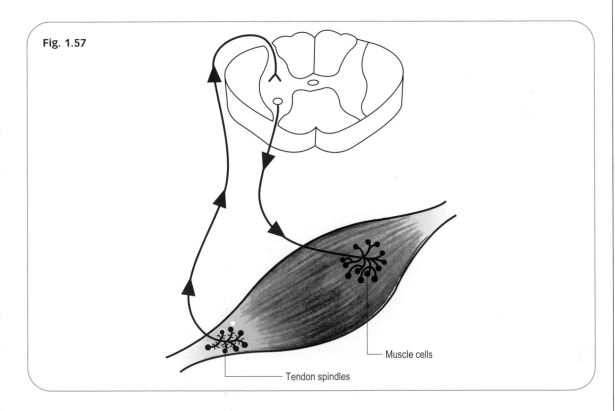

Fig. 1.57

Muscle cells

Tendon spindles

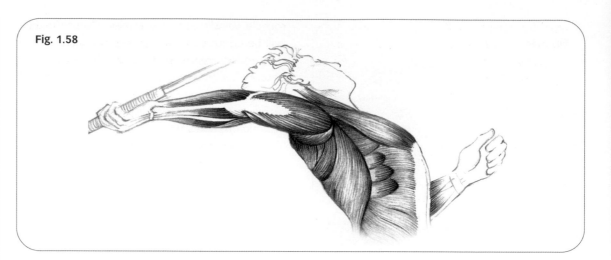

Fig. 1.58

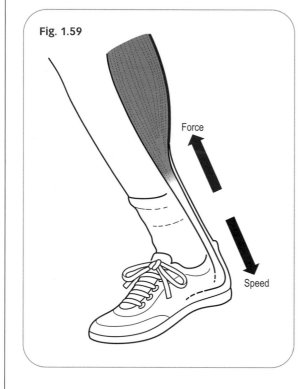

Fig. 1.59

Force

Speed

Around the joints and in the joint capsules are additional sensory cells that transmit information used to adjust movements and protect the body from injuries. Figure 1.60 shows three different nerve cells, each of them having the specific task of sending information.

Pacinian corpuscles are sensitive to pressure. Ruffini's corpuscles are sensitive to position and speed. The third type are the so-called free nerve endings that are sensitive to pain. These have a strong representation in capsules, in perimysium around muscles, and in periosteum around bones. A kick on the tibia (shin bone) can cause severe and immediate pain, but if nothing

forwards in making the hit. The tendon organs measure the force that acts on the tendon and send signals that reduce the contracting force, because the force is so great that there is a risk of a rupture in the tendon. If the force from the muscle reduces too far, the heel will sink down towards the floor, and the player might miss the shuttle cock and lose a point. But what is that compared to a ruptured Achilles tendon (heel tendon)?

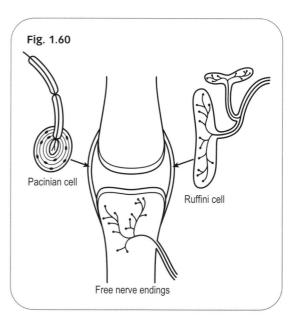

Fig. 1.60

Pacinian cell

Ruffini cell

Free nerve endings

is injured the pain will disappear after as little as 10 seconds. A soccer player who is writhing in evident pain but stands up right away when the game starts again and starts to run normally doesn't have to be a case for Hollywood.

Motor unit

In order to judge the value of different strengthening exercises, one should be aware of the following.

A muscle is made up of a large number of muscle cells. These are an integral part of so-called motor units. Each motor unit also includes a nerve cell, which has connections to the brain and which branches off into fine filaments terminating in the muscle (Figure 1.61). Each of these branches terminates in a single muscle cell. The number of cells in a motor unit depends on the degree of precision required from them. The muscles that are responsible for the movement of the eye, for example, contain 5 to 10 cells in each motor unit. By comparison, the gluteus maximus (large muscle that forms the fleshy part of the buttock) (p. 54) is estimated to contain several thousand cells in each unit.

When the motor unit is put to work, all the cells that comprise it contract. If a muscle is compelled to contract with a certain force, the work is carried out by a certain number of motor units. If the force of contraction is to increase, more motor units have to be engaged. The same motor units are thought to be used for coping with a light load, and other additional

units are engaged thereafter when the load increases. It is always specialized motor units that are ultimately engaged when the work load becomes maximal.

Light work-loads exercise only the muscle cells in the motor units that are first engaged. If we want to exercise an entire muscle, we must subject it to maximum stress.

There are two different types of muscle cells: slow (type-I) and fast (type-II). The slow cells are characterized by being supplied with energy via oxygen in the blood. The fast cells use mainly the energy stored in the muscle (as glycogen), which can be transformed into mechanical energy without oxygen. A by-product of this process is lactic acid. Different people have different percentage distributions of these cell types. The usual proportions are 50% type-I cells and 50% type-II cells. There are, however, great individual differences. Moreover, different muscles have different compositions of cell types.

In recent years it has been revealed that it would be appropriate to divide the type-II cells into two subgroups: type-IIa and type-IIb (Figure 1.62). Special training can change the character of type-IIa cells in such a way that

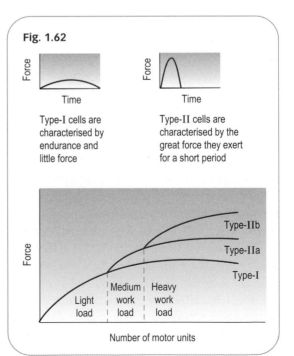

Fig. 1.62

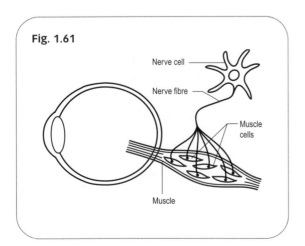

Fig. 1.61

they become more like type-I cells, i.e. they are supplied with energy via oxygen and are thus capable of greater endurance.

It has been shown that when a muscle is required to exert force the cell types are engaged in the order, type-I cells, type-IIa cells and, finally, type-IIb cells. When little force is required, only the type-I cells are used (see Figure 1.62, bottom).

Type-IIa cells have many of the best qualities of type-I and type-IIb cells, i.e. great strength and good endurance. Knowledge of the above is important when we wish to train for a special type of sporting event. However, it should be made clear that the designation 'slow' does not mean that the muscle cells contract so slowly that they do not contribute to the movements of sports. Such 'fast' movements as a golf swing and tennis smash are actually very slow compared with the speed with which the type-I cells contract.

In recent years, a large number of studies, concerning different muscles' composition of slow and fast muscle cells, have been conducted. In these studies, researchers have attempted to describe how different cells change during different types of training. The question whether fast cells can be transformed to slow cells through a certain type of training or vice versa is one that is hard to answer. There are great difficulties in finding answers to these kinds of questions. We know that different types of fibres are found in different parts of the muscle, which means that when a muscle biopsy is conducted (a small piece of the muscle is cut out and analysed using different chemical methods) to determine if it is type-I or type-II, at a certain spot or at a certain depth, we get a particular result. If we take the test at another spot, we get another result even though the test is taken in the same muscle. A biopsy is a rather large operation in a muscle and therefore there are ethical reasons why we don't conduct several tests in a muscle. It is also difficult to know if possible changes to the fibre composition, after for example, prolonged endurance training, are due to the effects of training or due to the fact that the test is taken a little deeper or to the side of the spot where it was taken before. Type-I cells (slow) are controlled by a particular type of nerve

cell and type-II cells are controlled by another type; therefore it cannot be said that a slow cell is completely transformed into a fast cell. In fact, the nerve cells do not change. It is presumed, however, that after a very long period of power training, muscle cells that work with a good oxygen supply can adapt to operate without a full supply of oxygen. In that way they assume some of the characteristics of type-II cells. It is also presumed that type-II cells can be taught to work at a more persistent production of energy with help from an improved blood flow and therefore oxygen supply. As a result there will be less lactic acid production, which means that the cell can work for a longer period of time before signs of exhaustion occur as mentioned above. Type-II cells can be divided into type-IIa and type-IIb. Type-IIa cells have proved to be the most adaptable of the two when it comes to different types of training. Instead of looking for changes after specific training, it could be even more interesting to determine if inheritance of a particular distribution of cell types affects the predisposition for different types of physical activity.

Figure 1.63 illustrates the distribution of type-I cells in the muscles of different sportsmen. It can

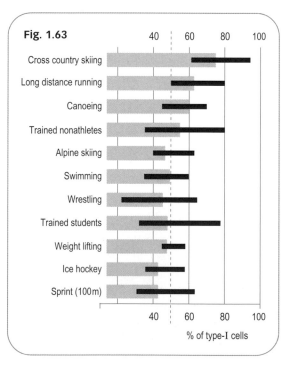

Fig. 1.63

% of type-I cells

be seen from the figure how the fibre type varies according to the sport undertaken. (The dark red bars represent the variation around the mean value.)

There is a clear bias for type-I cells in endurance sports and a bias for type-II cells in sports where the stress is on strength and speed.

The predisposition among people undertaking exercises at a non-elite level might depend on whether their muscles are suited for a particular activity or not. Some investigations have shown a relatively high correlation between a high percentage of type-I cells and a predisposition for running. Another correlation shows that the majority of people who undergo fitness training, have a high percentage of type-II cells. Figure 1.64A and B illustrate this point.

The question is, what causes what? Has an uneven distribution of cells affected the predisposition for a certain type of training or has the training affected the distribution of cells? From the discussion above it is tempting to think that hereditary factors are in operation in this area.

Training of different kinds changes the ability of muscle cells to perform work.

It is known with certainty that after prolonged work of relatively low intensity, the following changes occur in type-I cells:

1. The capillary net in the muscle, mainly around the type-I cells, increases. Thereby, the ability to supply the operating cells with oxygen and energy-providing substances also increases.
2. The number and size of mitochondria in the cell increase. Thereby, the ability to produce energy increases at the required pace.

   (ATP, adenosine triphosphate, is a high-energy compound produced by the mitochondria and is needed as a source of energy for muscle cells to contract.)
3. The number of repetitions possible with loads at a certain submaximal level increases. (A person can perform the same movement many more times.)
4. The size of the cells changes very little or not at all, and thereby the force exerted by the cell does not increase (there is no increase in strength).

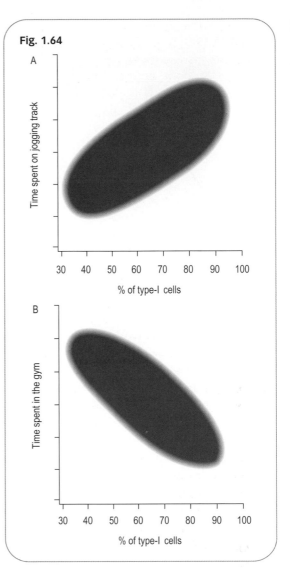

Fig. 1.64

A

Time spent on jogging track

% of type-I cells

B

Time spent in the gym

% of type-I cells

Training with heavy loads affects mainly type-II cells. The main changes are that:

1. The size (the cross-section) of the cells increases. (More force can be produced. There is an increase in strength.) The increase of the cross-sectional area depends on the fact that more fibrils are created in the cell. (There is the same number of cells in the muscle as before.)
2. The cell's ability to work without oxygen increases. (A person can work harder, and for a longer period of time, before too much lactic acid prevents effective work being done.)

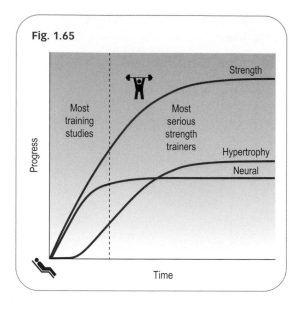

Fig. 1.65

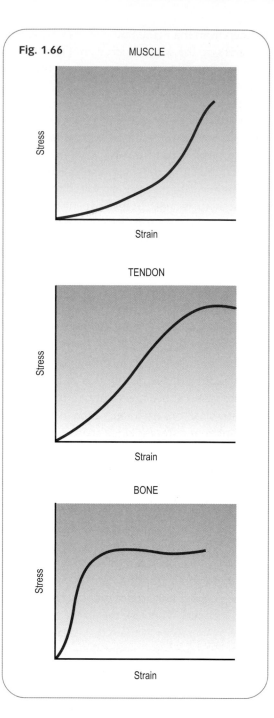

Fig. 1.66

When muscle cells work with heavier loads than normal the force generated increases (Figure 1.65). The increase in strength depends first on an improved cooperation between nerves and muscles (when you know the movement you will use the right muscles and more motor units) and secondly on greater muscle force (greater muscle cross-section) when the muscle does a contraction.

As well as the muscle cells undergoing these changes the tendons and the fibrous tissue adapt and acquire the ability to manage heavier loads. Muscle cells grow faster than tendons, which can cause problems in the tendons and their attachments to the bones. If a person exercises intensively during a short period of time soreness or decreased agility are warning signals that should be taken seriously. Training will also result in an increase in the density of the skeleton. As a result the skeleton becomes more stable and provides an extra protection against osteoporosis, which often causes broken bones among older people.

The curves in Figure 1.66 show how muscles, tendons and bones change their length (strain) when they are subjected to pulling forces (stress).

The curves illustrated in Figure 1.66 show that the muscle, which is elastic, reacts with a large extension to a relatively small stress. The tendons are more resistant and the bones make small

adjustments. With heavy loads, on the other hand, both bones and tendons can be stretched considerably before breakages or rupture occur. The muscle, on the contrary, becomes progressively stiffer as the load increases, before it ruptures. It is speculated that at heavy loads the system will be struck primarily by a ruptured muscle instead of a ruptured tendon or a broken

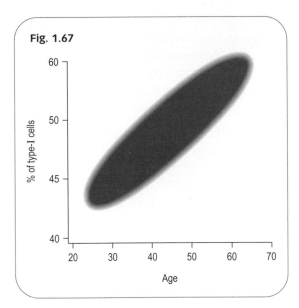

Fig. 1.67

y-axis: % of type-I cells (40, 45, 50, 60)
x-axis: Age (20, 30, 40, 50, 60, 70)

bone. A ruptured muscle often heals faster and, seen from that perspective, is the preferable of the three types of injury.

It has recently been proved that adaptation of muscles, tendons and the skeleton to regular training can be achieved at a very advanced age. A group consisting of nine people with an average age of 90 years trained their leg-extensor muscles over 8 weeks. The increase in strength for the group was fully 170%. By using the muscles, the ageing process is delayed. The muscle cells that degenerate because of age are mainly type-IIb. The curve in Figure 1.67 shows how the composition of cells in one of the knee extensors, the vastus lateralis (external vast thigh muscle) changes with advancing age.

E. Flexibility training
Different types of stretching

In order to maintain the natural flexibility of the joints and reduce the risk of injury in athletics, the training programme should always contain suitable and correctly executed flexibility exercises. A muscle that is only trained for strength becomes shorter. This, in turn, means that its range of movement is restricted which, in practice, decreases its ability to utilize its increased force resources correctly. Exercises that are designed to train the strength of a group of muscles, should always be followed by stretching exercises for the same muscle group.

Elastic stretching is used here to denote the activity of rhythmically swinging an arm or leg towards its most extreme position. This swinging action has nothing to do with stretching the muscles. Elastic stretching has been used, and should be used, when warming and limbering up.

On the other hand, stretching exercises are those designed to lengthen the muscle groups used as effectively as possible, which in turn increases the range of motion in the joints. Thus, both stretching exercises and elastic stretching exercises are used to promote general agility.

Assume that a person wants to increase the range of movement of his arm so that he can draw it back as far as possible (swimmer, thrower, gymnast).

(A) If the arm is swiftly swung back (Figure 1.68), it could perhaps reach position *a*. What happens is that the muscles situated behind the shoulder give the arm its speed, but the arm is halted before it reaches an outer position. This halting is caused by the spindles in the muscles at the front of the joint and endings in the joint itself that send warning signals to the CNS (central nervous system). The CNS, in turn, sends

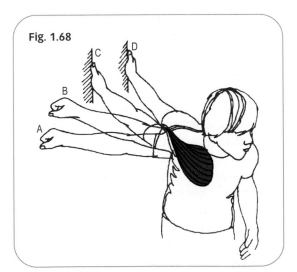

Fig. 1.68

contraction signals to the same muscles in order to prevent injury of the cells. Instead of stretching, the muscles on the front side of the joint are forced to contract to protect themselves and the joint. This type of elastic stretching may produce eccentric strength but it certainly does not train flexibility. When elastic stretching is performed forcefully by a person who is not warmed-up, the risk of minor ruptures is obvious. However, easy elastic stretching is a good way of toning the muscle.

(B) If, instead, the arm is slowly drawn back as far as it will go, the position it reaches will generally be farther than that of the swinging arm described above. Just how far back depends on the suppleness of the muscles at the front of the joint, and the strength of the muscles that pull from the back of the joint. This method is called active stretching. Work is actively being done by the antagonists (the muscles on the other side of the joint) to the muscles we want to stretch. However, we try as far as possible to relax the actual muscles that are to be stretched.

(C) In passive stretching the arm is forced backwards further with the help of external forces (i.e. not the muscles at the back of the shoulder). This could be done, for example, with the aid of a friend, or the hand could be held against a wall and pressed backwards, thereby utilizing the force of the legs. Passive stretching is always more effective than active stretching in reaching the outermost position.

(D) The best results will be obtained, however, by first extending the arm as far as possible by the passive-stretching method. (The muscle group that is to be stretched should be as relaxed as possible.) Next, try to contract the muscle group for a few seconds (6 s) while the external force (friend, legs, wall) prevents any movement occurring at the joint. The muscle tension is thus static, which implies that the muscle belly is somewhat shortened and the collagenous fibres of the tendons are somewhat extended.

By relaxing again (2–4 s), after which passive stretching is again exercised, the arm could reach even farther.

The method of contracting a muscle with the aim of increasing its ability to stretch is called the PNF method (Proprioceptive Neuromuscular Facilitation). The PNF method is used by physiotherapists when they train an injured muscle in an effort to restore its natural length. It is also called the contraction–relaxation–stretching method. In Figure 1.69, the arms are used as an effective form of resistance when the muscle contracts.

Contraction affects the tendon organs of the muscle with the result that they send out inhibitory signals to the muscles during the ensuing relaxation. The limb should be close to the outermost position the whole time, and any movements should be slow and easy so that the muscle spindles are discouraged from sending contraction signals to the muscle.

Figure 1.70A shows what happens when one tries to stretch a contracted muscle. The external force acting on it affects only the muscle cells, and consequently only minor muscle ruptures can result.

Figure 1.70B shows that when the muscle is relaxed, it is the fibres of the connective tissue that are stretched. Connective tissue is more rigid and can resist swift stresses (jerks, elastic

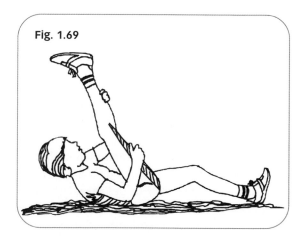

Fig. 1.69

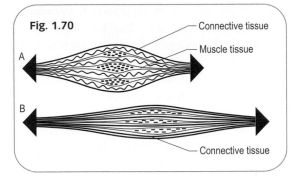

Fig. 1.70
- Connective tissue
- Muscle tissue
- Connective tissue

A

B

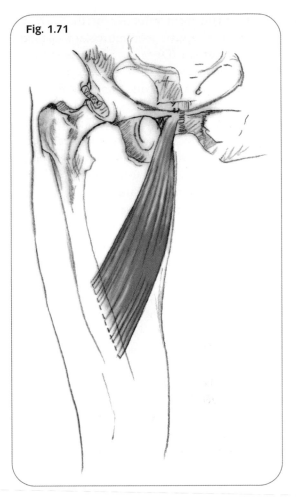

Fig. 1.71

stretching) but yields to prolonged stress (remain in the outermost position for about 30 s).

Examples of flexibility development

The example below is designed to demonstrate further how a muscle group can be stretched effectively, i.e. how the flexibility of a particular joint can be improved. Good flexibility in the hip joint is of great importance to nearly all athletes. The group of muscles that are easily injured and which impede effective movement patterns, are the muscles of the groin (the adductors). These originate from the pubis (pubic bone) and are inserted into the femur (thigh bone) (Figure 1.71) (see p. 56). When sitting on the floor with the soles of the feet together (Figure 1.72) and as close as possible to the body, it will be seen that the length of the groin muscles will determine just how far the knees can be pressed to the floor.

When, in the same position, the knees are bounced up and down, the activity corresponds to that described in (A) on p. 31. Further, if the knees are pulled down using the muscles of the outer side of the hip (abductors, p. 54), the activity corresponds to the method described in (B) on p. 32, i.e. active stretching of the groin muscles. Pressing the knees down with the elbows corresponds to the method described in (C) on p. 32, i.e. passive stretching of the groin

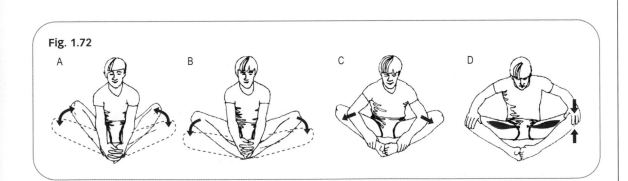

Fig. 1.72

A   B   C   D

muscles. The most effective method, i.e. the PNF (proprioceptive neuromuscular facilitation) method (method (D) on p. 32), is practised in the following way.

Press down with your hands holding back with your knees (about 6 s), relax (2 s), press down with your hands again (10 s), hold back once again (6 s), relax (2 s) and finally press with your hands for about 10 s with relaxed groin muscles.

The rectus femoris (straight thigh muscle), (p. 64) can be stretched using the PNF method in the following way. Take your foot in your hand. Bend your knee maximally and try to keep your hip as straight as possible. Next, try to extend the knee joint while holding back with your hand for about 6 s (the rectus femoris thus contracts statically) (Figure 1.73).

Next, relax for 2 s. Then slowly press your hip forward a little and stand still for about 10 s. Repeat this several times.

It has been shown that the number of muscle injuries in, for example, soccer has been radically reduced when flexibility exercises are introduced as a regular part of the training programme. A properly executed stretching exercise following the PNF method, takes about 20 s. A soccer player should perhaps work through five different muscle groups, about

three times on each training session, in order to obtain good results: $20 \times 5 \times 3 = 300$ s. Thus, more than 5 minutes are required each time he trains. Many trainers claim that they have no time for flexibility training; but better knowledge of how to perform this type of training, as well as its benefits, should dispel such arguments. However, a prerequisite for this is that the trainer acquires in-depth knowledge of the origin, insertion and function of muscles.

Suitable positions for stretching exercises are shown in Chapter 7. Before looking into that, we have to learn more about the most important muscles (Chapters 3–5).

F. Strength training

It is customary to distinguish between different types of strength (Figure 1.74).

In addition, dynamic strength is divided into concentric and eccentric strength (p. 19).

The majority of cells in the body are capable of reproducing themselves. This, however, does not apply to striated muscle cells. Their numbers are almost entirely determined by genes. When training for strength, the muscle cells are thus not increased in number. Instead, there is an increase in the number of myosin and actin filaments, which are responsible for muscle contraction. Consequently, enlargement of cells takes place. Like the majority of cell types, the muscle cells follow the principle of overcompensation. According to this principle, training breaks down parts of the stressed structures.

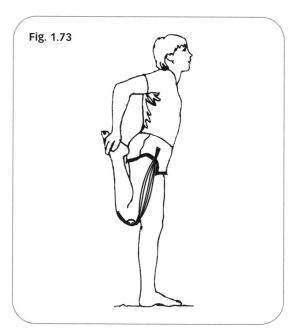

Fig. 1.73

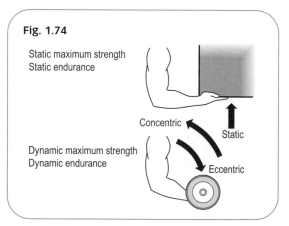

Fig. 1.74

Static maximum strength
Static endurance

Concentric

Static

Dynamic maximum strength
Dynamic endurance

Eccentric

The body compensates for this by producing new fibrils, the number of which is somewhat greater than the number of fibrils broken down. The athlete should begin the next training session at the time when overcompensation has reached a maximum (Figure 1.75).

When the training sessions are too close together, or the training too vigorous without extra long pauses, the regeneration of fibrils never reaches the previous level. The athlete thus slowly wears down the body – becomes 'overtrained'.

As a general rule, we can say that recovery normally takes 24–48 hours (after extremely vigorous training, about 72 h). Thus, an athlete should train relatively vigorously three times a week in order to increase strength quickly.

Strength decline is first noticeable after 5–6 days without training. About one session a week should therefore suffice for an athlete to maintain the strength that is already there.

As mentioned earlier, youths should not train with loads exceeding their own bodyweight before or during puberty. Because children younger than 11 or 12 years find complicated movements difficult, they should avoid exercises demanding coordination. Training with light weights aims at accustoming young people to the equipment as well as developing the correct technique.

On the basis of what has been said about motor units (p. 27), strength should be developed by using heavy work loads (all the motor units must be activated). A common target for an athlete is 80–95% of what can be maximally managed. In this way the ability to work at a dynamic maximum is improved. If the athlete wishes to improve dynamic endurance, loads that correspond to 20–25% of maximal capacity should be worked with. Endurance training has the effect of decreasing both the maximal strength and speed of the muscle group in question. Training for speed is undertaken with a work load of 50–80% of the maximum that can be managed by the athlete.

There are two main types of muscle cell: white and red. They have received their names from the colour they assume when they are specially treated to be examined under the microscope. The fast muscle cells (type-II) described on p. 27, are the white cells, and the slow muscle cells (type-I) are the red. White muscle cells contain many actin and myosin filaments (see p. 13). Red muscle cells contain slightly fewer but, on the other hand, have more energy-supplying components.

These conditions result in strong, fast white cells that tire quickly; and red cells that are characterized first and foremost by their endurance. Both red and white fibres are contained in the same muscle. A muscle's composition is determined by genes, but it can, in part, 'be changed' by specific training (p. 27).

Different sporting events require different types of strength, so athletes and trainers should choose exercises with care. Weight-lifting is dependent on strong, fast muscles. Weight-lifting training should, therefore, involve few exercises that are designed for dynamic endurance. It has been shown that pure endurance training considerably reduces both the strength and speed of the muscles used.

The concepts 'sets' and 'repetitions' (reps) are often used in descriptions of strength development. A set contains a particular exercise that is repeated a certain number of times. A set can, for example, consist of six consecutive repetitions (various scientific investigations indicate that the quickest increase in strength is acquired with six reps). Several reps with a light work load promote endurance. Fewer reps with a heavier work load develop maximal strength.

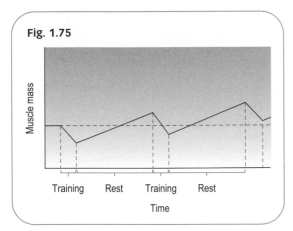

Fig. 1.75

Muscle mass

Training   Rest   Training   Rest

Time

If we take, as an example, an exercise that strengthens the pectoralis major (the greater chest muscle), then a weight should be chosen that can be lifted and lowered six times with slightly bent arms (to avoid straining the elbow joint). This should be followed by a period of rest (2–3 minutes) (Figure 1.76). During the pause a completely different muscle group – e.g. the quadriceps femoris (four-headed thigh muscle) – can be developed in the same way. The exercise for the pectoralis major is then repeated, i.e. using a second set with its six reps. An instruction that reads 'five sets × six reps' means a total of 30 lifts with five 2–3 minute pauses after each set.

The work load can be varied, as the amount of arm flexion varies (see the mechanics section on levers, p. 40). A muscle is stronger when it works eccentrically than when it works concentrically. This is easily verified by slowly lifting a weight; it feels easier to lower than to lift. If the aim is to develop eccentric strength, the athlete should keep the arms almost straight while lowering weights, and bend them while lifting.

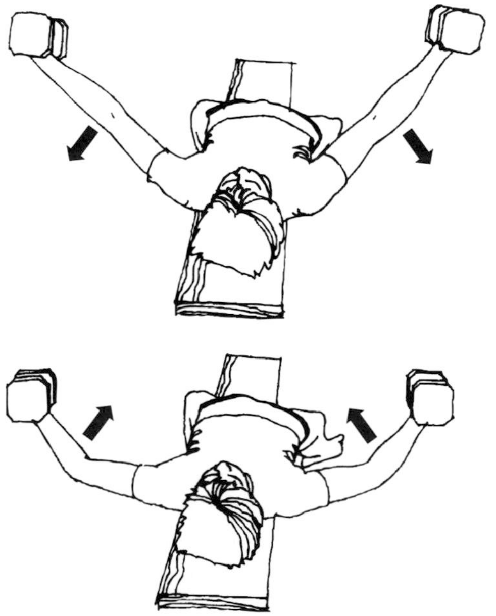

A curve that presents an approximation of the number of times a movement can be performed has been constructed experimentally (Figure 1.77). This number depends on the ratio of work load to the maximal load the muscle group in question can manage.

Another curve (Rhomert's curve) (Figure 1.78) shows how many minutes an isometric contraction can take if it falls short of the isometric maximum of the muscle group.

A method for quickly building up the strength of muscles is the so-called pyramid system. For each set the work load (weights) is increased and the number of reps is decreased so that the effort exerted in the final set is maximal.

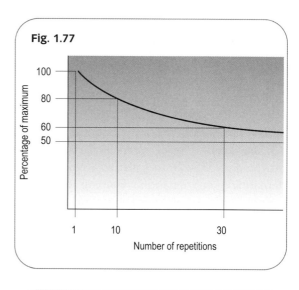

Fig. 1.77

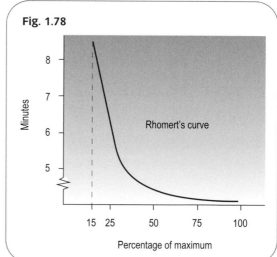

Fig. 1.78

Fig. 1.76

Set 1: Six reps with 70% of the maximum weight that can be lifted.

Set 2: Five reps with 75% of the maximum weight that can be lifted.

Set 3: Four reps with 80% of the maximum weight that can be lifted.

Set 4: Three reps with 85% of the maximum weight that can be lifted.

Set 5: Two reps with 90% of the maximum weight that can be lifted.

Set 6: One reps with 95–100% of the maximum weight that can be lifted.

It should be pointed out that the strength of muscles increases faster than the strength of tendons, ligaments and cartilage. Extremely vigorous training can, therefore, injure muscle attachments and joints.

The table below (Figure 1.79) gives approximate work loads together with the number of times exercises should be carried out in order to develop different types of strength. Exercises for developing strength are described in each section of the book where the anatomy of different parts of the body is dealt with (e.g. the knee joint, p. 67).

You will learn more about strength in Chapter 2. At the end of Chapters 3–5 you can read about special training exercises for specific muscle groups.

Fig. 1.79

	Endurance	Speed	Maximal strength
% of max.	25-50	50-80	80-100
Number or reps	more than 40	approx. 10	1-6
Number of sets	5	4	3

Basic rules of mechanics

Chapter 2

Torque

In order to understand how the skeleton is constructed and how the muscles affect a particular part of the body, we must familiarize ourselves with certain properties of force as well as what is meant by the concept 'moment of force' or 'torque'.

In Figure 2.1 a force (*F*) is represented by an arrow indicating its magnitude and direction.

If an object weighs 5 kg, it is said that the gravitational force acting on it is 50 newtons (50 N) (Figure 2.2).

If a force is applied to a body at a certain distance (*l*) from a certain point (Figure 2.3), the force may cause a certain angular motion at that point. This tendency towards angular motion is called the moment of force (or torque) and is represented by *M*. The moment of force is calculated by multiplying the magnitude of the

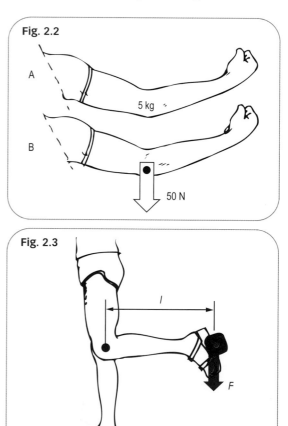

Fig. 2.2

A

5 kg

B

50 N

Fig. 2.3

l

F

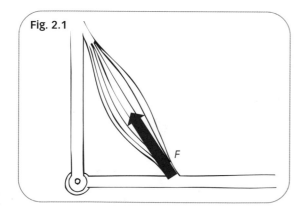

Fig. 2.1

F

force (F) by the distance (l) between the force and the point. Thus:

$$M = F \times l$$

The magnitude of the moment of force tells us just how much the object is striving to rotate. Thus, the moment of force is a quantity that depends on two factors at the same time; it should be noted that the same force can have different rotating effects depending on its point of application.

In the examples represented in Figure 2.4, the force applied is the same but the moment of force varies such that it is least in Example 1, and greatest in Example 3. Suppose that the force applied is 50 N and the respective distances are: $l_1 = 0.2$ m, $l_2 = 0.3$ m and $l_3 = 0.5$ m. The moment of force is then calculated according to the formula:

$$M = F \times l$$

The results 10, 15 and 25 Nm (Newton metres) show how much the wrench handle tends to turn.

The moment of force of 25 Nm can be obtained in many different ways. An alternative to Example 3 would be to apply a force of 100 N at a distance of 0.25 m from the bolt (Figure 2.5); $M_4 = 100 \times 0.25 = 25$ Nm.

Example 5. If a mass (m) of 5 kg is placed 2 m from the fulcrum of a seesaw, the moment of force with respect to that point would equal 100 Nm, i.e. $M = 50 \times 2 = 100$ Nm (Figure 2.6).

Example 6. The moment of force of 100 Nm can also be achieved by placing a 10 kg load 1 m from the fulcrum (Figure 2.7).

$$M = 100 \times 1 = 100 \text{ Nm.}$$

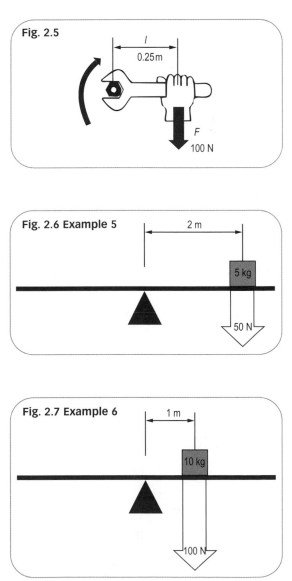

Fig. 2.5

0.25m

F
100 N

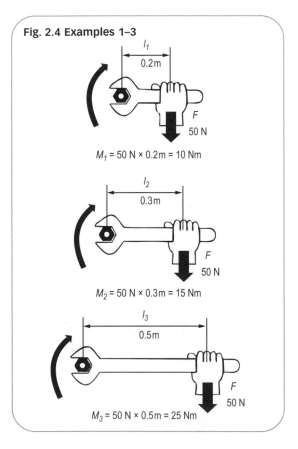

Fig. 2.4 Examples 1–3

l_1
0.2m

F
50 N

$M_1 = 50 \text{ N} \times 0.2\text{m} = 10 \text{ Nm}$

l_2
0.3m

F
50 N

$M_2 = 50 \text{ N} \times 0.3\text{m} = 15 \text{ Nm}$

l_3
0.5m

F
50 N

$M_3 = 50 \text{ N} \times 0.5\text{m} = 25 \text{ Nm}$

Fig. 2.6 Example 5

2 m

5 kg

50 N

Fig. 2.7 Example 6

1 m

10 kg

100 N

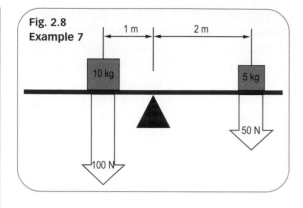

Fig. 2.8
Example 7

1 m

2 m

10 kg

5 kg

50 N

100 N

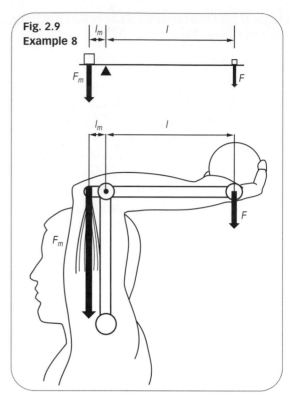

Fig. 2.9
Example 8

l_m

l

F_m

F

l_m

l

F_m

F

Example 7. If weights are placed at different distances on each side of the seesaw's centre as in Figure 2.8, then the seesaw is balanced. The moments cancel each other out (seesaw principle). $100 \times 1 = 50 \times 2$.

Similar reasoning can be applied to the way in which muscles affect different parts of the body.

Example 8.

F_m = Muscle force.

l_m = The distance between the muscle's lever arm and the centre of the joint.

F = The force of gravity acting on the ball.

l = Distance to the centre of the joint.

The elbow joint (Figure 2.9) can be compared with a seesaw where the external force (F) acts on one side and the internal force (F_m)

acts on the other. The arm is held still if $F_m \times l_m = F \times l$.

Example 9. The body in Figure 2.10 is in equilibrium when $F_m \times l_m = F \times l$. If $F_m \times l_m$ is greater than $F \times l$, the body accelerates upwards (rises

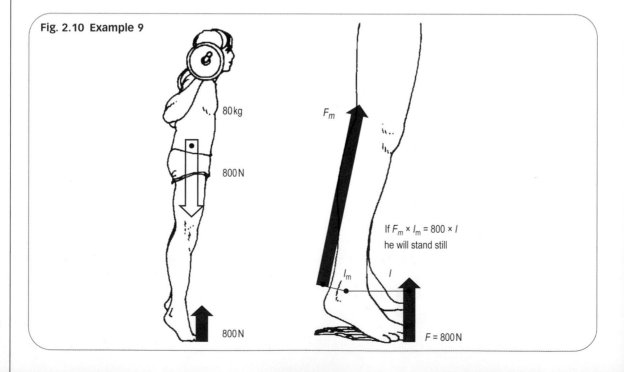

Fig. 2.10 Example 9

80 kg

800 N

800 N

F_m

If $F_m \times l_m = 800 \times l$
he will stand still

l_m

l

$F = 800\,N$

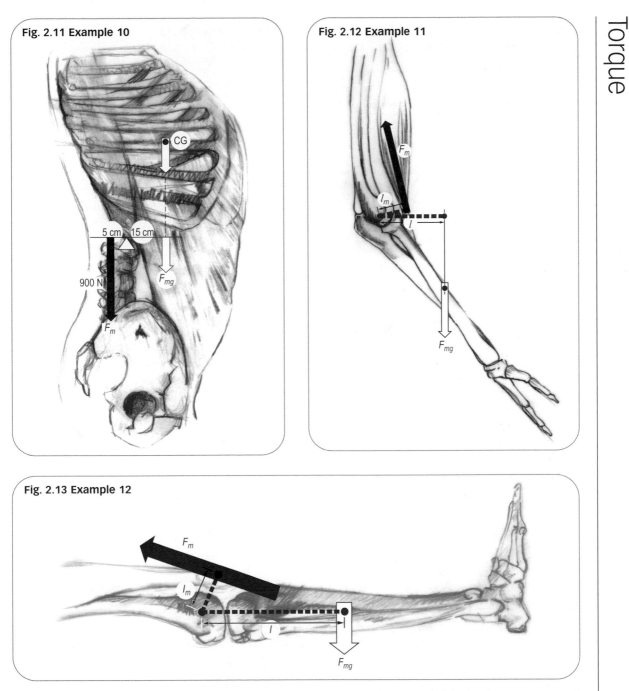

Fig. 2.11 Example 10

CG

5 cm 15 cm

900 N

F_m

F_{mg}

Fig. 2.12 Example 11

F_m

l_m

l

F_{mg}

Fig. 2.13 Example 12

F_m

l_m

l

l

F_{mg}

even further on its toes). If $F_m \times l_m$ is less than $F \times l$, the body will not be able to hold its position and will sink. The body + barbell has a mass of 80 kg.

Example 10. The weight of the trunk (30 kg) is counterbalanced by the traction force of the back muscles. If the centre of gravity (CG) of the trunk lies three times as far in front of the vertebrae as the back muscles lie behind them, then the traction force of the back muscles must be three times greater than the trunk weight (Figure 2.11).

In general, the part of the body in question will accelerate (start rotating) in the direction where the moment of force is greater.

Examples 11–14. In Figures 2.12–2.14, the force of gravity (F_{mg}) and the force of the muscle are both located on the same side of the joint, but pull in different directions. $F_m \times l_m = F_{mg} \times l$ can be applied to all three.

In Figure 2.15, the forearm (1 kg) is acted on by a gravitational force of 10 N. If the centre of

Fig. 2.14 Example 13

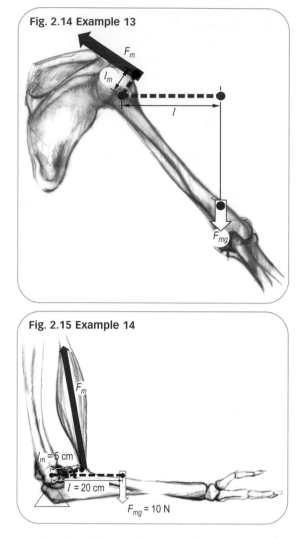

F_m

l_m

l

F_{mg}

Fig. 2.15 Example 14

F_m

$l_m = 5$ cm

$l = 20$ cm

$F_{mg} = 10$ N

Fig. 2.16 Example 15

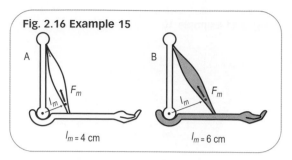

A

F_m

l_m

$l_m = 4$ cm

B

F_m

l_m

$l_m = 6$ cm

The muscle of person B is attached at a point further from the joint, which means that the perpendicular distance to the muscle force is, for example, 6 cm when the elbow is bent at a 90° angle.

If the muscle force (F_m) is equal for A and B, the moment of force (strength) will be 50% greater for B than for A. Thus, B is stronger than A.

If the muscle is contracted by 3 cm in both cases the forearm of A will move through a greater angle than the forearm of B. Thus, A has faster movement than B (Figure 2.17). This proves to be true if it is not carrying a heavy object.

The ability of muscle to develop force (F_m) can be influenced by strength training, but a muscle's attachments cannot be changed (Figure 2.17). In other words, we are constructed in such a way that we are particularly suited to certain activities and less suited to others – at least so far as top performance is concerned.

Tendon and ligament forces are passive (Figure 2.18). This means that they are brought

gravity lies 20 cm from the joint, then the moment of force will be equal to 10 × 20 Ncm (Newton centimetres). If the muscle that bends the elbow is attached at a point 5 cm from the joint, then F_m × 5 must equal 10 × 20 if the arm is to be held still (F_m must then equal 40 N).

The diagrams illustrate different types of joints and the way in which the body has solved the problem of resisting (or creating) movements.

If the point of insertion of the arm's most important flexor differs in two people, then these two people will differ greatly in the strength and speed of movement of their arms.

Example 15. Suppose the muscle of person A is attached at a point that gives a lever arm of 4 cm when the elbow is bent at a 90° angle (Figure 2.16).

Fig. 2.17

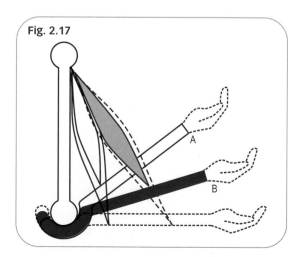

A

B

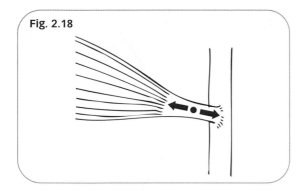

Fig. 2.18

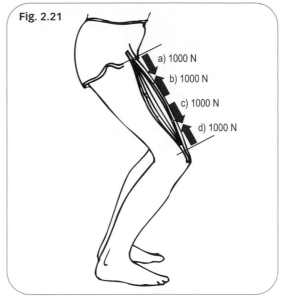

Fig. 2.21

a) 1000 N
b) 1000 N
c) 1000 N
d) 1000 N

about by external forces (Figure 2.19) or by the muscles (Figure 2.20).

If we consider a small part of a taut tendon, we can understand that it strives to resist a stretch. Thus, we can draw an arrow indicating force either in the direction of muscle pull or in the direction of tendon (muscle attachment) resistance (see Figure 2.18).

Suppose a person is standing with knees slightly bent and that one of his knee extensors is contracted with a force of 1000 N (Figure 2.21). The force acting on its origin is then 1000 N (a)

and is directed towards the knee. A force of 1000 N (d) is acting on the patella (kneecap) and is directed towards the thigh. A bundle of connective tissue somewhere in the muscle stretches with a force of 1000 N (b and c). The tension in the tendon extending between the patella and the tibia (shin bone) is also about 1000 N. The force acting on the apex of the patella and the tendon's attachment are both 1000 N (see Figure 2.22).

The above explanations of how to draw force arrows and how to calculate muscle forces with

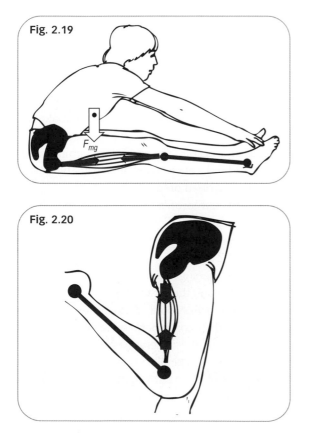

Fig. 2.19

F_{mg}

Fig. 2.20

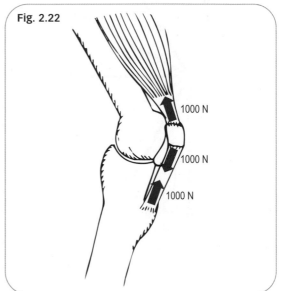

Fig. 2.22

1000 N

1000 N

1000 N

the aid of the seesaw principle, are applied to the descriptions of the body's structure in the following chapters.

Before the body's different muscles and joints are described in more detail we will, with the help of the concept of torque, look at what occurs during strength training. Some of the most common muscles and the most frequently used training machines will be used as examples.

If you do a biceps curl (lift a dumbbell as in Figure 2.23), there will be an external torque on the elbow joint equal to the weight of the dumbbell multiplied by the perpendicular distance from the joint to the line of direction for the force of gravity. This distance varies during the movement from 0 cm to a maximum of 30 cm when the lower arm passes the horizontal. The distance then decreases to 0 cm again when the dumbbell is held directly above the elbow joint.

This can be described in a diagram showing the torque that the flexor muscles of the arm must manage in order to be able to perform the movement slowly. This kind of curve is called a torque curve (or actual torque).

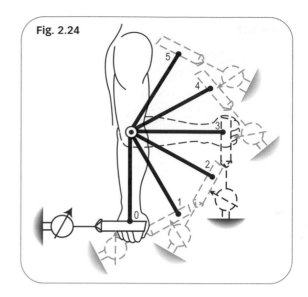

Fig. 2.24

By measuring the flexor muscles' maximum capacity in different parts of the moving area in Figure 2.24, a curve called the muscles' strength profile can be drawn.

For the flexor muscles in the elbow joint, the strength profile is measured using apparatus such as a dynamometer that, when operated, entails using the whole forearm as a lever. The maximum force that can be developed is also measured by the machine.

The force multiplied by the length of the forearm, in each position, will be the maximal torque. To do this isometrically is quite easy. You will just need a good dynamometer. To make the same measurement when the muscle is contracting at a certain speed is more complicated. You would then have to use an isokinetic device which is described on p. 20.

The strength profile for the flexor muscles in the elbow in terms of isometric strength (or slow movements) approximates to that shown in Figure 2.25.

A strengthening exercise is beneficial if the torque curve and the strength profile of the muscle correspond fairly well. With, for example, the biceps curl, they correspond quite well. One can describe what is happening if you adjust the weight of the dumbbell so that the torque curve lies slightly below the strength profile during the greater part of the arm movement. The area between the curves in Figure 2.25 indicates how

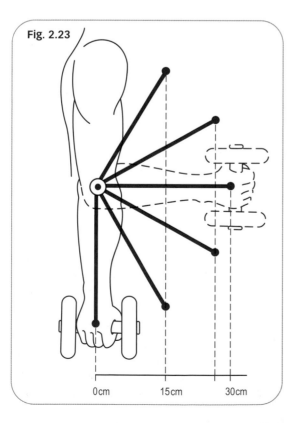

Fig. 2.23

0cm   15cm   30cm

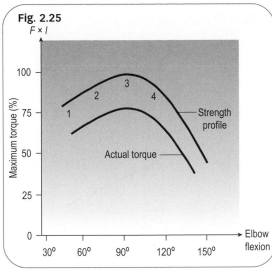

Fig. 2.25

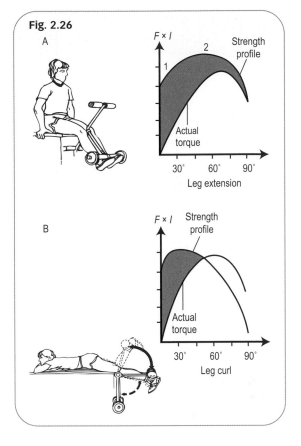

Fig. 2.26

much extra strength a person has in every part of the movement. The numbers 1–4 in Figure 2.24 refer to the same numbers as in Figure 2.25. A frequently used model is to work with 80% of maximum strength and perform six repetitions (reps). If the curves correspond well the exercise will be efficient in all parts of the movement. If the curves do not correspond so well the exercise will be inefficient and difficult to perform. The result of the training will be negative, with injury as a possible consequence.

Apparatus such as that in Figures 2.26A and B give a torque that varies during the exercise (see the accompanying graphs).

If the apparatus is used for the knee-extensor muscles, whose strength profile is like that shown in Figure 2.26A, it functions well. If it is used for the flexor muscles in the knee, with a strength profile as shown in Figure 2.26B, there will be some problems. The torque will become greater and greater at the same time as the muscle group becomes weaker and weaker. The exercise will be too easy at the beginning and impossible at the end. The result will be that the speed of the movement will be too high at the start of the exercise, since the load is too light, but appropriate in the mid-phase of the exercise when torque and strength are more or less equivalent. In the end the exerciser is forced to release the load without finishing the move-

ment. The effect of the training is not particularly beneficial.

The new types of weight machines have, to a large extent, adapted to problems of this type. Nowadays, asymmetric gear-wheels are used to produce torque curves that correspond with a particular muscle group's strength profile. Suppose that you want a machine that adapts as closely as possible to the strength of the knee extensors (Figure 2.27).

You choose the desired weight and with a chain and a gear-wheel you transfer the force to the arm of the apparatus that loads the lower leg. The gear-wheel can be constructed in such a way that the torque varies in much the same way as the strength profile for the working muscle group. You just have to make sure that the distance from the centre of the gear-wheel is correct in every part of the movement. If Fl_1 equals the value at point 1 in the strength profile in Figure 2.26A you have to work at 100%

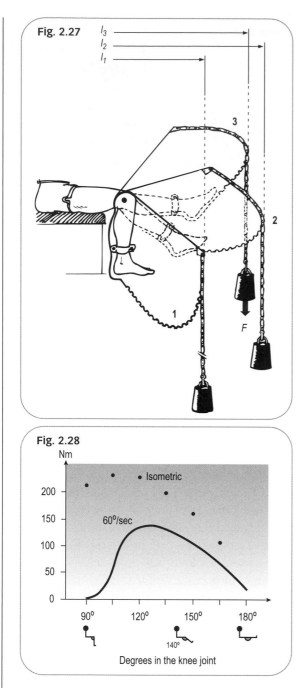

Fig. 2.27

Fig. 2.28

Nm

• Isometric

200

150   60°/sec

100

50

0

90°   120°   150°   180°

140°

Degrees in the knee joint

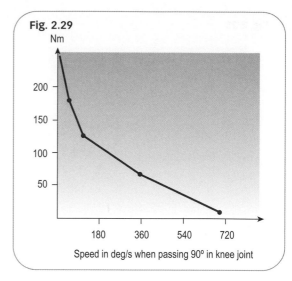

Fig. 2.29

Nm

200

150

100

50

180   360   540   720

Speed in deg/s when passing 90° in knee joint

statically in six different positions and at a speed of 60°/s. The measurements were taken using an isokinetic dynamometer (see Figure 1.45) where the movement starts at a knee angle of 90° and the knee is extended until it is straight.

Figure 2.29 shows how much torque a person can produce starting at a knee angle less than 90° and with a rotational velocity that varies between 0 and 720°/s.

Definition of Work (*W*) and Power (*P*)

Work

If you lift an object that weighs 10 kg from the floor and place it on a table that is 1 m high, you have performed work equivalent to 100 Nm (Figure 2.30).

Work (*W*) is defined as Force (*F*) multiplied by the distance over which the force is operating.

$$W = F \times l$$

In our example, a 10 kg object is acted on by the force of gravity, i.e. 10×9.81 Newtons. The quantity 9.81 N/kg is the conversion factor that is used to calculate the gravitational force of an object. This is represented by the symbol g. Most of the time, if you are only discussing principles that are not dependent on exact values, the figure of 9.81 is rounded up to 10 in order to make calculations simpler. Generally, the force of gravity acting on an object of mass (m) is mg N.

capacity to be able to lift the weight. Fl_2 corresponds to 100% for another knee angle (point (2) in Figure 2.26A). You have to work at maximum in that position too, and so on. If you now lower the weight to 80% of your ability you will have a perfectly adjusted machine for strength development of your knee-extensor muscles.

The graph in Figure 2.28 shows how large a torque the knee-extensor muscles can produce

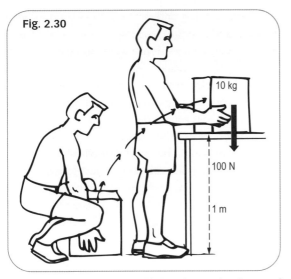

Fig. 2.30

In our case with the 10 kg object the force of gravity will be:

10×9.81 or $10 \times 10 = 100$ N.

The distance that the object was lifted was 1.0 m. The total work then became $100 \times 1.0 = 100$ Nm. The energy your muscles have produced when lifting the object has been transformed into Potential energy. Work is also performed when you are pulling an object along the ground (Figure 2.31). You pull with a force that overcomes the force of friction between the object and the ground's surface. The energy your muscles have produced raises the temperature of the object and the ground. This kind of energy is called Thermal energy. The work that is performed also depends on the distance (l) over which the object is pulled. The work done can be defined as $W = F \times l$, where F = force of friction and l = distance.

Below you can compare four different situations where the same amount of work is carried out.

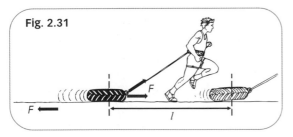

Fig. 2.31

1. For the bench press shown in Figure 2.32 the work performed is $300 \times 0.40 = 120$ Nm.

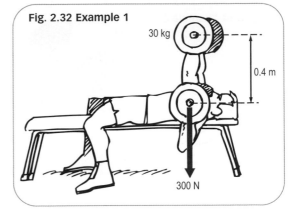

Fig. 2.32 Example 1

2. Doing a step up on a stair-case (Figure 2.33) the work performed is $600 \times 0.20 = 120$ Nm.

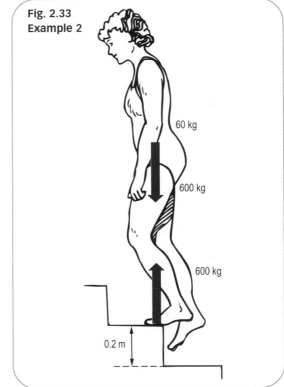

Fig. 2.33 Example 2

3. If you are lying on a leg-extension machine (see Figure 2.34) the work performed will be $mg \times h$. You will not take into account a possible force of friction when the 'wagon' glides along the rails. If the load is 60 kg and the distance in height 0.2 m the work performed will be:

$$W = F \times l = m \times g \times h = 60 \times 9.81 \times 0.20$$
$$W \approx 600 \times 0.20 = 120 \text{ Nm}$$

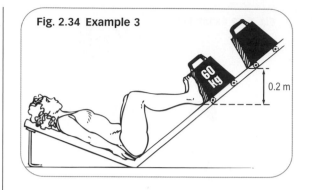

Fig. 2.34 Example 3

60 kg

0.2 m

4. When the pedals on a testing bike are turned through a single gyration, the wheel will turn a certain distance depending on how the gear wheel is constructed. The wheel is then loaded to give a force of friction of the desired magnitude. It is possible to pedals at a rate corresponding to a work output of 120Nm. Suppose that a single gyration of the pedals makes the wheel turn 6 meters (depending on the radius of the wheel); if you then set the force of friction at 20 N the performed work will be:

$$W = F \times l = 20 \times 6 = 120 \text{ Nm}.$$

Work has also been done when you increase the speed of an object. The amount of work depends on the mass (m) and the gain in speed (v) the object has received. The formula to calculate the work done is:

$$W = \frac{1}{2} \times mv^2$$

The energy is called Kinetic energy.

Suppose the girl in Figure 2.34 'kicks' so hard on the 60 kg wagon that it leaves her feet with the velocity 3 m/s. The total amount of work will then be 120 Nm due to the height she lifts the wagon + 270 Nm due to kinetic energy.

$$\frac{1}{2} \times mv^2 = \frac{1}{2} \times 60 \times 3^2 = 30 \times 9 = 270 \text{ Nm}$$

Physicists say that produced energy can be transformed to different forms (but not destroyed). When a muscle contracts the energy usually appears as some combination of warmth (raised body temperature), potential energy (you have lifted something) and kinetic energy (you have speeded up something).

There is a big difference between endurance training and strength training. In endurance training relatively light loads are used, and the goal is to increase the muscles' capacity for prolonged work. The physiologists can then examine how much work is performed and thereby know how much oxygen is being used and therefore how much blood the heart must pump to the working muscles. They find that all oxygen transportation functions are being developed. After endurance training, where the pumping load is between 60% and 80% of the heart's maximal capacity, it is possible to achieve results such as:

1. Stronger heart
2. More blood pumped for every heart beat
3. Increased blood volume
4. Better oxygenated blood
5. Tighter capillary net in the muscles
6. More mitochondria (energy producers) in both types of muscle cells
7. Increased ability of the muscles to utilize the oxygen

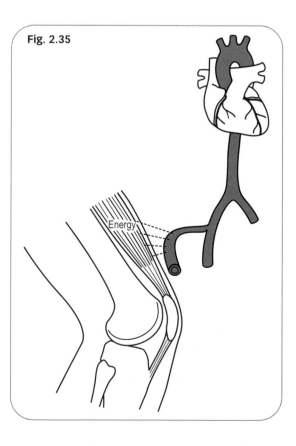

Fig. 2.35

Energy

Without the latter effect in the type-II cells the lactic acid level increases (Figure 2.35).

Power

Physicists and physiologists, when dealing with work ($F \times l$), normally take into account the time taken for the work to be performed. If a certain amount of work is performed over 5 minutes the heart will naturally pump faster compared with the same work being done over 10 or 15 minutes. To be able to include how fast work is performed the term Power is used. Power (P) is defined as work (W) per unit time (t).

$$P = W/t$$

The unit for work is the Newton metre (Nm). The unit used here for time is seconds (s). The unit for power then becomes Newton metre/second (Nm/s), which is also known as the Watt (W).

To test a person's physical status, one usually uses a test bike where the load is set on, for example, 150 W, 200 W or 300 W, all depending on the physical status of the person. The goal is to work with about 150–170 heart beats per minute to be able to manage the test. The person must also be able to work steadily for an extended time period without any major changes occurring – the person has thereby achieved 'steady state'. Using detailed tables you can calculate retrospectively the maximum oxygen uptake per kilogram body weight and unit time for the tested person.

For development of strength using heavy loads (see p. 37), which also increases muscle volume, work performance and power output are not usually taken into account. Instead, the focus is on how large the torque is and how many repetitions you can make.

Figure 2.36 gives an approximate correlation of how many reps you can make in relation to maximum capacity. This approximate correlation has been the basis of guidelines for different training models. When you talk about so-called speed training the loads are around 60% of maximum for the person doing the

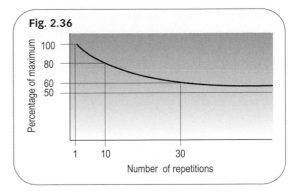

Fig. 2.36

training. One reason could be that the muscle has maximal power development at approximately 60% of maximum strength (torque). This can be determined if you measure, with two photo cells, the speed with which a person, for example, pushes up a barbell under various loads.

If a person pushes up 5 kg a distance of 0.5 m in 0.2 s, the power will be ($P = (F \times l)/t$):

$$P = (50 \times 0.5)/0.2 = 125 \text{ W}$$

If the same person pushes up 10 kg, the time might increase to 0.25 s, which gives a power of:

$$P = (100 \times 0.5)/0.25 = 200 \text{ W}$$

At loads close to a person's maximum, the tempo will be slow, resulting in low power.

In an investigation of three different muscle groups (Figure 2.37), power values were

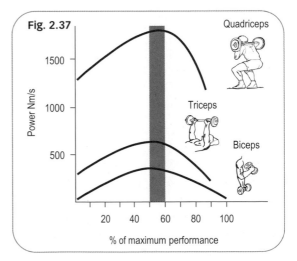

Fig. 2.37

determined at loads calculated in relation to the test person's maximal performance in every exercise.

For all three muscle groups, maximal power was achieved when the load was around 60% of maximal strength. In other words, if you work with 60% of your maximal strength and maintain a high tempo you probably improve your 'explosivity' in the most effective way.

Chapter 3

Anatomy and function of the leg

In order to analyse different types of movement correctly, we must first study the anatomy of the area concerned. Here, we will examine the origin, insertion and function of the larger muscles. In addition, we will look at the joints' potentials for movement and their limitations.

A. The hip

The majority of muscles responsible for moving the hip joint originate from the pelvis; some originate from the spinal column. Some of them also pass over the knee joint. Thus, we must acquaint ourselves with the parts of the skeleton shown in Figure 3.1 (anterior view).

The pelvis is the collective name given to a ring formed by the two hip bones and the sacrum. The sacrum consists of five vertebrae, which are fused together in the adult to form a wedge-shaped bone. Four terminal vertebrae are fused in the same way to form the coccyx (tail bone).

The hip bone (Figure 3.2; lateral view) has developed from three separate centres of ossification, which is why the following distinction is made:

1. Ilium (haunch bone).
2. Ischium.
3. Pubis (pubic bone).

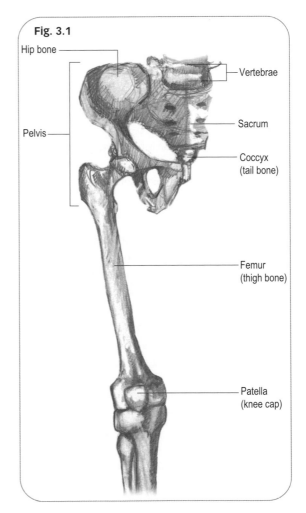

Fig. 3.1

Hip bone

Pelvis

Vertebrae

Sacrum

Coccyx (tail bone)

Femur (thigh bone)

Patella (knee cap)

Fig. 3.2

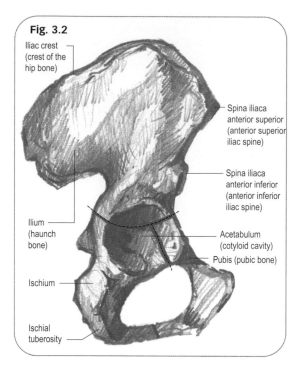

Iliac crest (crest of the hip bone)

Spina iliaca anterior superior (anterior superior iliac spine)

Spina iliaca anterior inferior (anterior inferior iliac spine)

Ilium (haunch bone)

Acetabulum (cotyloid cavity)

Pubis (pubic bone)

Ischium

Ischial tuberosity

Fig. 3.3

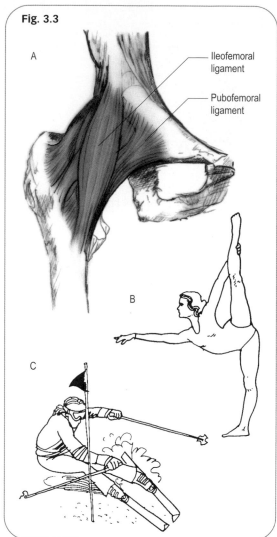

A

Ileofemoral ligament

Pubofemoral ligament

B

C

All the cavities, outgrowths and spines have different names. Those that are directly connected with important muscles are given here:

1. Spina iliaca anterior superior (anterior superior iliac spine).
2. Spina iliaca anterior inferior (anterior inferior iliac spine).
3. Acetabulum (cotyloid cavity).
4. Ischial tuberosity.
5. Iliac crest (crest of the hip bone).

The hip joint is a so-called ball and socket joint, which means that it can move in all directions (p. 9). There are certain extra-capsular structures that give strength to the joint and, in particular, prevent the leg from swinging outwards and backwards. Backward swinging is impeded by the powerful ligament that is attached to the iliac part of the hip bone and that passes downwards to the femur (thigh bone) – the iliofemoral ligament. Outward swinging is restricted by the pubofemoral ligament (Figure 3.3A; anterior view).

Figure 3.3B and C above demonstrate actions that demand great flexibility of the hip.

It has not been shown that any injury is sustained when a person stretches in the directions mentioned above. If, on the other hand, a person compensates for a poor ability to swing his leg backwards by overstretching the lumbar region of his back, he would in probability be literally 'making a rod for his own back'. Overstretching the lumbar area often leads to pain of a more or less serious character.

Details of the femur and the knee region are shown in Figure 3.4.

The patella (kneecap) (Figure 3.5) has a base that is directed upwards and an apex that points downwards. The inside of the patella is covered with a 6–7 mm thick layer of cartilage whose surface articulates with the cartilage-covered condyles of the femur.

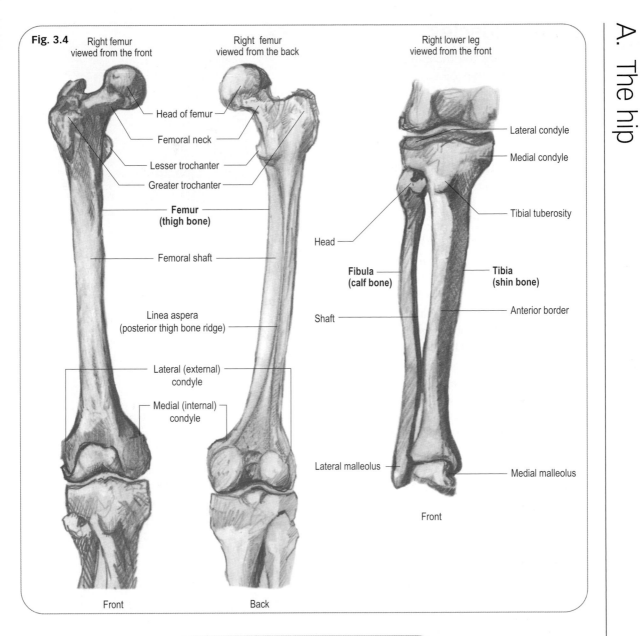

Fig. 3.4

Right femur viewed from the front

Right femur viewed from the back

Right lower leg viewed from the front

Head of femur

Femoral neck

Lesser trochanter

Greater trochanter

Femur (thigh bone)

Femoral shaft

Linea aspera (posterior thigh bone ridge)

Lateral (external) condyle

Medial (internal) condyle

Lateral condyle

Medial condyle

Tibial tuberosity

Head

Fibula (calf bone)

Tibia (shin bone)

Anterior border

Shaft

Lateral malleolus

Medial malleolus

Front

Front

Back

Front

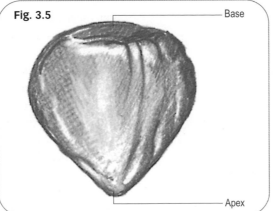

Fig. 3.5

Base

Apex

B. Hip muscles

The following are the most important muscles that pass over the hip joint:

1. Buttock muscles.
2. Groin muscles.
3. Hip flexors.

1. Buttock muscles (the abductors)

1. Gluteus maximus (large buttock muscle).
2. Gluteus medius (intermediate buttock muscle).
3. Gluteus minimus (small buttock muscle).

Two of the three muscles are attached to the greater trochanter. The gluteus medius and minimus buttock muscles have such a large area of origin that they can move the femur (thigh bone) in all directions except inward towards the midline of the body (adduction). These muscles are activated during walking and running. They have the important task of stabilizing the hip joint when the corresponding foot alone is in contact with the ground. This stabilization is necessary in order to prevent the upper body from falling to the opposite side.

The buttock muscles are subjected to great stress when a person runs uphill (the gluteus maximus muscle is responsible for the powerful backward drive of the leg) or downhill (gluteus medius and minimus stabilize the hip). The gluteus medius

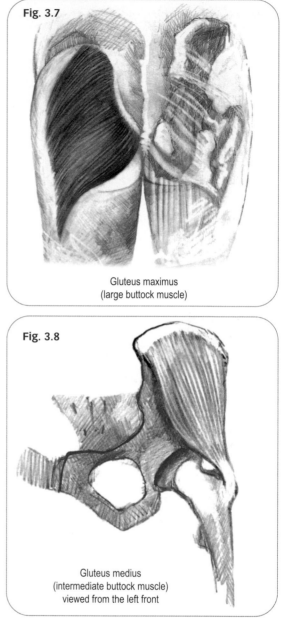

Fig. 3.7

Gluteus maximus
(large buttock muscle)

Fig. 3.8

Gluteus medius
(intermediate buttock muscle)
viewed from the left front

and minimus then work eccentrically, i.e. they restrain the upper body so that it does not fold inwards at every step (Figure 3.6). Figures 3.7–3.9 show the gluteus maximus, gluteus medius and gluteus minimus respectively.

Examples of exercises for the buttock muscles: running; jumping on one leg; and, while standing on one leg, lowering and raising the opposite side of the pelvis. Further exercises for the gluteus medius and minimus are: (A) lying on one side and lifting the upper leg and (B) lifting the upper part of the body as far as possible while the legs are fixed (Figure 3.10).

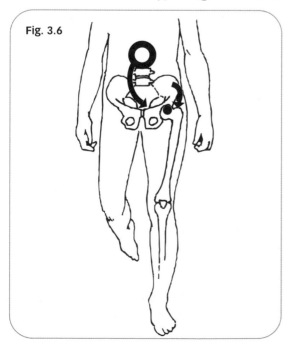

Fig. 3.6

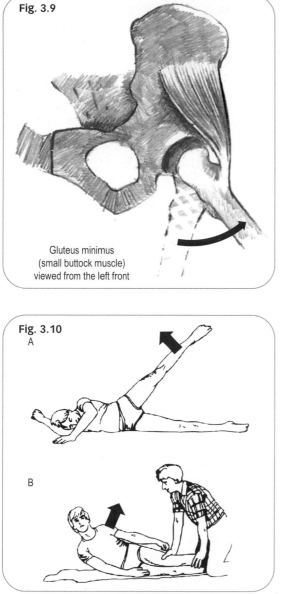

Fig. 3.9

Gluteus minimus
(small buttock muscle)
viewed from the left front

Fig. 3.11

Gluteus maximus
(large buttock muscle)

Iliotibial tract

Fig. 3.10

A

B

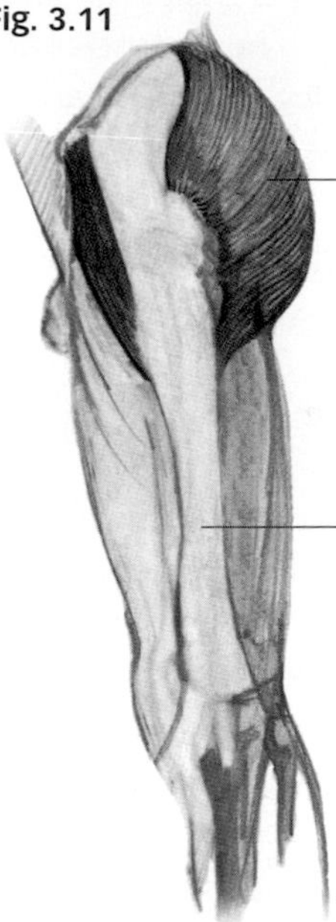

Fig. 3.12

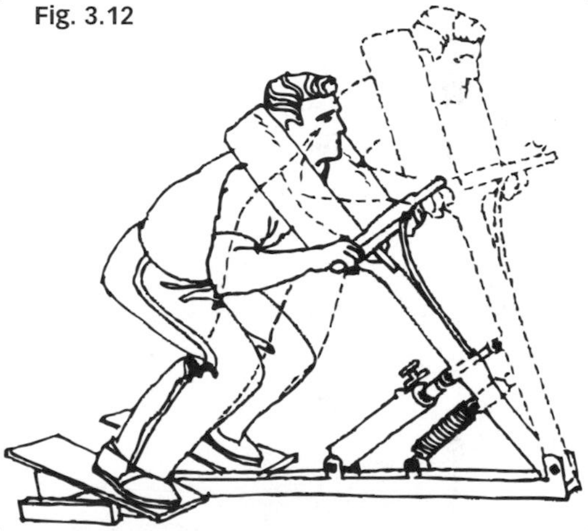

The gluteus maximus is used to swing the leg backwards powerfully, and it can help to straighten the knee. This is possible because a part of the muscle is attached to the surface of the femur (at the gluteal tuberosity), which straightens the hip, and a part is inserted into a very strong, thick tendon band on the outer side of the thigh (iliotibial tract) (Figure 3.11; lateral view). This tendon band passes, in turn, in front of the axis of motion of the knee and is inserted into the lateral tibial condyle (external condyle of the skin bone). The tendon band is felt as a flat 3–4 cm wide tendon on the outside of the thigh directly above the knee joint.

The gluteus maximus can work with greater force if the body is bent forward at the hip. This is because the distance between its origin and insertion becomes greater (see p. 17). Figure 3.12 shows how the more force a person needs, the further forward he must bend at the hip. The best movements for training the gluteus maximus are those that simultaneously engage the knee and hip extensors.

The muscles that take part in swinging the leg backwards (hip extension) are – besides the

55

gluteus maximus – those muscles originating from the ischial tuberosity. These muscles are all inserted into the lower leg which means that they flex the knee joint (see p. 69).

2. The groin muscles

These adductor muscles swing the leg towards the midline of the body. They have received their names according to their area of origin, size and appearance.

All these muscles originate mainly from the pubis (pubic bone) and are inserted into the posterior surface of the femur (thigh bone) via the roughened ridge that extends along the length of its shaft (linea aspera). Figures 3.13, 3.14 and 3.15 show anterior views of the pectineus ('comb' muscle), gracilis (slender thigh muscle) and the adductor longus (long adductor muscle) respectively. Figures 3.16 and 3.17 show anterior views of the adductor magnus (large adductor muscle) and adductor brevis (short adductor) muscles. These muscles work powerfully when, in running, the foot leaves the ground and begins to swing forwards. During the forward swing, the leg rotates outwards in relation to the hip. This can be accomplished because the adductor muscles are inserted into the posterior surface of the femur. Such overexertion as occurs in the

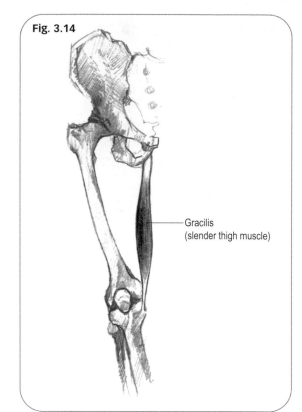

Fig. 3.14

Gracilis
(slender thigh muscle)

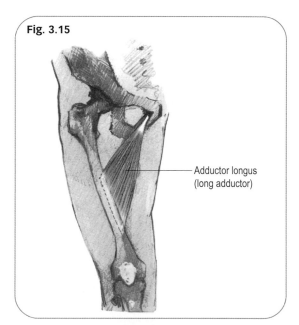

Fig. 3.15

Adductor longus
(long adductor)

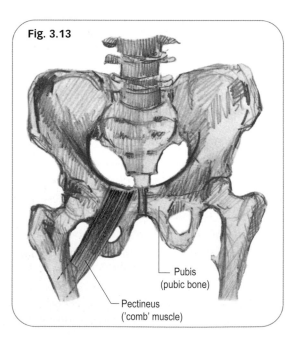

Fig. 3.13

Pubis
(pubic bone)

Pectineus
('comb' muscle)

forceful movements of broad side kicks in football, bringing the free leg forward in skating, tough sprint training, etc., leads to discomfort in the muscle's area of origin (groin injuries). Groin

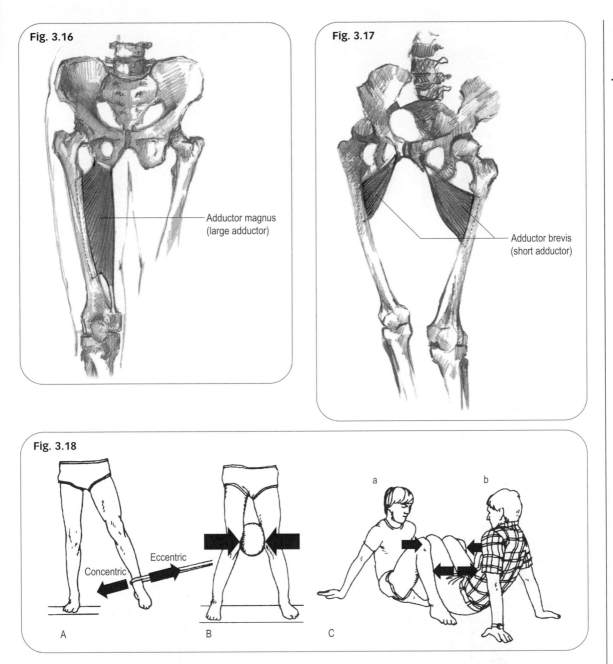

Fig. 3.16

Adductor magnus
(large adductor)

Fig. 3.17

Adductor brevis
(short adductor)

Fig. 3.18

Concentric   Eccentric

A   B   C

a   b

injuries can be avoided by developing muscular strength and, more importantly, flexibility (p. 31). Some strength-developing exercises are shown in Figure 3.18. This figure (A) illustrates how concentric training involves bringing the legs together, whereas eccentric training involves slowly drawing one leg away from the other, and (B) how static training can be performed by compressing a ball with both knees. The exercise in (C) trains the adductors of person a and the abductors of person b.

Outward rotation is effected by a number of small muscles that originate from the inner parts of the pelvis (Figure 3.19A; lateral view). They pass behind the femur and are inserted into its outer surface at the greater trochanter. They are used a great deal in activities such as ice-skating. Figure 3.19B shows an example of dynamic training of the outward rotators. Figure 3.19C shows an example of static training of the outward rotators; this involves lying on your stomach and trying to squash a ball with your feet.

Fig. 3.19

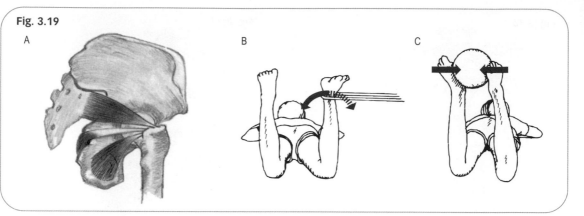

A   B   C

3. Hip flexors

The iliacus (haunch muscle) and psoas major (great lumbar muscle) (Figure 3.20; anterior view) are responsible for powerful flexion at the hip joint. They have different points of origin (a and b), but a common insertion point (c). They are often described under the collective name of the iliopsoas.

The following can occur when the iliopsoas contracts:

1. If the legs are fixed (Figure 3.21), the trunk will move towards them as, for example, in the last phase of a sit-up.
2. If the trunk is fixed (Figure 3.22), the legs will move towards it as, for example, when hanging from a bar and trying to bring the knees up towards the chest.

The iliopsoas is incomparably the most powerful hip flexor. It is forcefully engaged in the examples shown in Figure 3.23.

It is not necessary to train the iliopsoas for everyday use since it is sufficiently trained in

Fig. 3.21

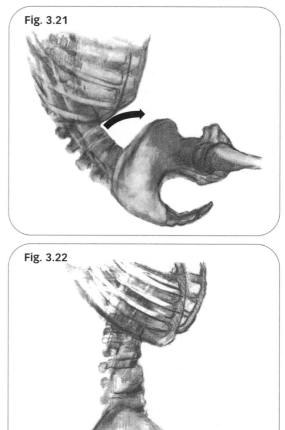

Fig. 3.20

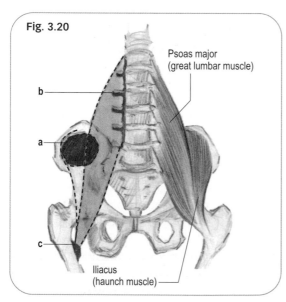

Psoas major
(great lumbar muscle)

b

a

c

Iliacus
(haunch muscle)

Fig. 3.22

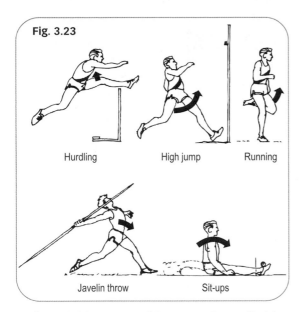

Fig. 3.23

Hurdling High jump Running

Javelin throw Sit-ups

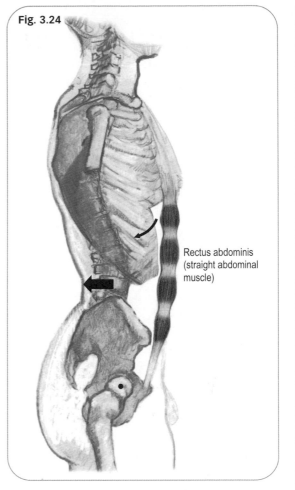

Fig. 3.24

Rectus abdominis (straight abdominal muscle)

such activities as walking, running, climbing stairs, etc. Athletes must realize that the stress they subject this muscle group to when they train it for strength affects both the insertion and origin (e.g. lumbar vertebrae) to the same extent. Thus, the spine tends to sway forwards which subjects the discs between the vertebrae (p. 88) to great stress. This action is counteracted by the abdominal muscles, which hold the spine in place (Figure 3.24). The abdominal muscles are capable of correcting a sway of the lumbar spine by their contraction. Thus, the iliopsoas should not be subjected to greater stress than the abdominal muscles are capable of 'parrying'. Training ought to be aimed primarily at building up the abdominal muscles (p. 98).

After building up the abdominal muscles, the hip flexors can be specially trained. Here are some examples of exercise that specifically train the hip flexors (Figure 3.25A–F) of athletes whose abdominal muscles are well-trained. (Prophylactic training of the abdomen is dealt with on p. 100.)

Figure 3.25A. Sit-ups with bent knees. Weights (2 kg, 5 kg, …) may be held against the chest to increase the work load. The first three-quarters of the sit-up is pure abdominal muscle training. The rest of the movement concentrates on the hip joint and thus trains the iliopsoas for strength.

Figure 3.25B. If the legs are kept straight, then the exertion will be even greater due to the resistance offered by the muscles at the back of the thigh.

Figure 3.25C. Lie on a slanting plane or hang from a bar and lift your knees towards your hands, or

Figure 3.25D (for greater stress) lift your legs as high as possible, keeping them straight. For eccentric training, resist the movement on the way down.

Figure 3.25E. Stand by a wall and have a friend provide external resistance to your thigh as you try to lift your knee.

Figure 3.25F. Tie a band of rubber around your foot and pull your knee up in quick movements.

Figure 3.25G. The hip flexors can be trained statically in the following way. Lie on your back with a 90° angle at your hips and have a friend take a hold of the lower part of your shin. By making large movements in different directions, he should try to make you change the angle between your legs and upper body.

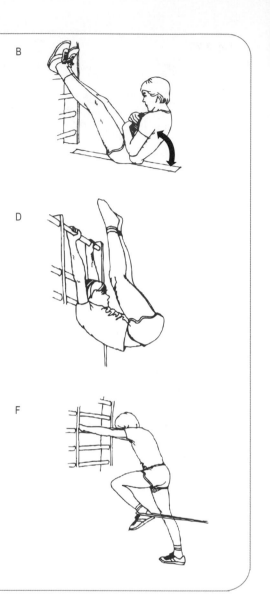
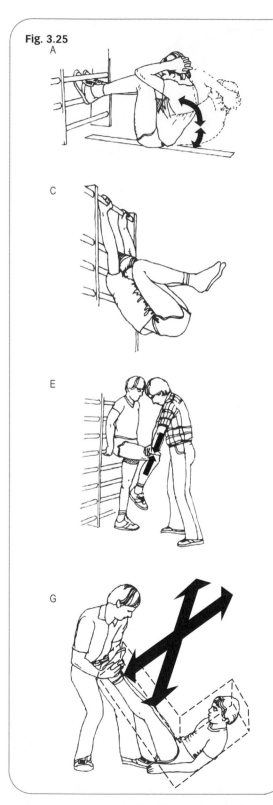

Fig. 3.25

In order to stretch the iliopsoas, the distance between its origin and insertion must be lengthened as much as possible while the muscles are relaxed. One way to stretch it is to kneel in the manner shown in Figure 3.26A, i.e. the stress is placed on the leg in front and the legs are separated as much as possible. If the iliopsoas is short and strong, but the muscles at the back of the thigh are weak, then the body tends to tip forwards at the pelvis. This leads to mild back-aches and a posture resembling that of a person with a 'beer belly'.

Another stretching exercise that has an effect on the iliopsoas is the following: stand on one leg and with your hand pull your free leg back behind an imagined line passing vertically through the centre of your body (Figure 3.26B). Let the backward movement take place at the

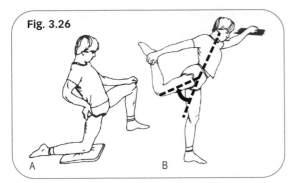

Fig. 3.26

hip and not in the lower back. Keep a wide angle at the knee joint, otherwise the movement will be resisted by another muscle, namely the rectus femoris (straight thigh muscle, p. 64).

A third stretching exercise is shown in Figure 3.27. A friend lifts your leg upwards and backwards as while holding your pelvis still at the same time (thereby blocking any movement of the lumbar spine). This exercise should only be carried out by people who have received their instructions from a medically qualified trainer.

The sartorius (tailor's muscle) is the longest muscle in the body (Figure 3.28). It extends from the spina iliaca anterior superior (anterior superior iliac spine) and passes down the thigh in a slightly S-shaped curve to the inner side of the knee where it is attached to the medial tibial condyle (internal condyle of the shin bone).

This muscle has so many different functions that it is difficult to place it in any particular muscle group. The tailor's muscle received its name from the fact that its functions allow a person to sit on a table with crossed legs as tailors once did. Thus, this muscle bends, abducts and rotates the hip outwards, and bends the knee and rotates the lower leg inwards.

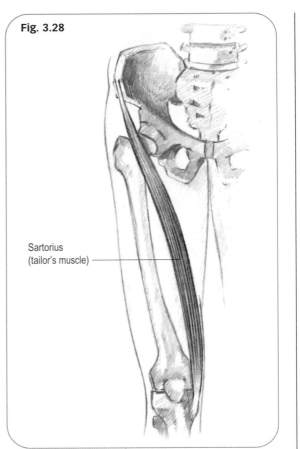

Fig. 3.28

Sartorius
(tailor's muscle)

C. The knee joint

The knee joint is a very complicated joint that needs detailed study. The movements produced at the knee joint are bending (flexing) and straightening (extending), and inward and outward rotation of the lower leg relative to the upper. The last-mentioned movements can only occur when the knee is bent. The more the knee is bent, the easier it is to rotate the lower leg and the foot. We can think of the knee as flexing either by (Figure 3.29):

1. the femur (thigh bone) rolling back on to the tibia (shin bone)(A) or by
2. the femur gliding on the same spot on the tibia (B).

In reality, both types of movement occur. Movement (A) takes place until the anterior cruciate (cross) ligament is completely stretched, after which movement (B) is brought into action.

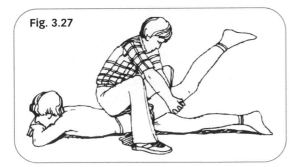

Fig. 3.27

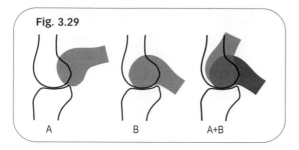

Fig. 3.29

Thus, the anterior cruciate ligament (Figure 3.30) prevents movements when the lower leg is moved forwards in relation to the thigh. A common injury in football is rupture of the anterior cruciate ligaments which can happen when a player's foot is blocked and the lower leg rotates inwards. The posterior cruciate ligament is injured when the lower leg is pressed backwards or when the knee is severely overstretched.

The function of the two side (or collateral) ligaments (Figure 3.31) is to prevent sideways bending of the knee. They are taut when the knee is stretched (A), and slack when the knee is bent (B). This means, for example, that the lower leg can be rotated outwards until the ligaments are again taut. The lower leg usually cannot rotate as much inwards as it can outwards because the cruciate ligaments in the joint twist around each other during inward rotation and thereby block the movement (see Figure 1.20).

The lower end of the femur is elliptical and the upper extremity of the tibia is flat. Therefore, there would be very little contact between their surfaces if the cartilage were not so thick and the so-called menisci were not shaped to receive the end of the femur. The undersides of the menisci are plain like the surface of the tibia. Consequently, the stress to which the knee is subjected can be distributed over a relatively large area. Most of the details in the knee can be seen in Figures 3.32–3.34.

In flexion and extension of the knee joint, the menisci glide to suit the form of the condyles of the femur. Because the medial meniscus fuses with the medial collateral ligament, it is very easily injured by being subjected to excessive stress while in 'strange' positions.

Injury to the menisci due to rotational strain on a bent weight-bearing knee is very common. If there is a sudden pitching in the knee joint during outward rotation of the lower leg, the medial ligament stretches and can thereby tear the meniscus, which is locked between the femur and tibia. Because of this, movements of the following type should be avoided: (A) crow hopping or walking like a duck and (B) lying in the hurdle position to train flexibility (Figure 3.35).

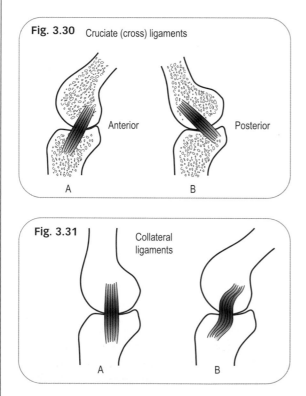

Fig. 3.30 Cruciate (cross) ligaments

Anterior

Posterior

A

B

Fig. 3.31

Collateral ligaments

A

B

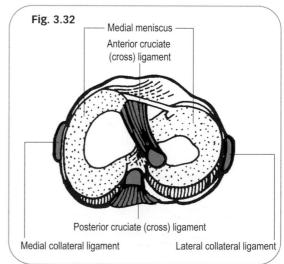

Fig. 3.32

Medial meniscus

Anterior cruciate (cross) ligament

Posterior cruciate (cross) ligament

Medial collateral ligament

Lateral collateral ligament

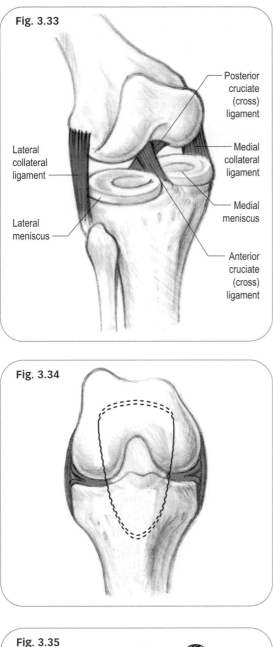

Fig. 3.33

Posterior cruciate (cross) ligament

Lateral collateral ligament

Medial collateral ligament

Medial meniscus

Lateral meniscus

Anterior cruciate (cross) ligament

Fig. 3.34

Fig. 3.35

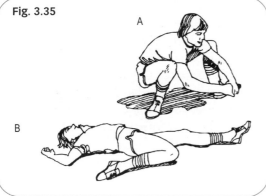

A

B

D. Muscles of the knee joint

Knee extensors

The rectus femoris (straight thigh muscle) originates from the pelvis and bends (flexes) the hip joint. It is inserted into the patella (kneecap) (Figure 3.36; lateral view) and can – via the powerful tendon that extends from the patella to the tibia (shin bone) – straighten the knee.

The way in which the rectus femoris works can be tested in the following way: stand on one leg with your body in the vertical plane and lift your free leg to the horizontal plane. Figure 3.37(B) shows that the muscle is maximally shortened in this position. Can you manage to lift your leg? Are the muscles at the back of your thigh (p. 70) flexible enough to allow you to straighten your leg? How long are you capable of holding that position? Very soon you will feel a smarting pain in the rectus femoris. The pain is a sign of the insufficient oxygen supply that quickly results from static activity. In Figure 3.37(A) the muscle is maximally stretched.

The position shown in Figure 3.37(A) is by far the best position for stretching the straight thigh muscle in accordance with the PNF (proprioceptive neuromuscular facilitation) method.

Three other large muscles are inserted into the knee joint. They are also extensors of the knee. They are termed the vastus muscles (vastus = extensive, far-reaching). The four diagrams of Figure 3.38 show the extensors in the right leg viewed from the front.

Origin and insertion:

A. The vastus intermedius (central vast thigh muscle) has its origin on a large area of the front of the shaft of the femur (thigh bone). The cells are rather short and it ends on a broad collagen sheet that reaches down to the patella.

B. The vastus lateralis (external vast thigh muscle) and vastus medialis (internal vast thigh muscle) start on the linea aspera (posterior thigh bone ridge). Most of the muscles cells go 180°, from the back of the shaft all the way round it, and attach to

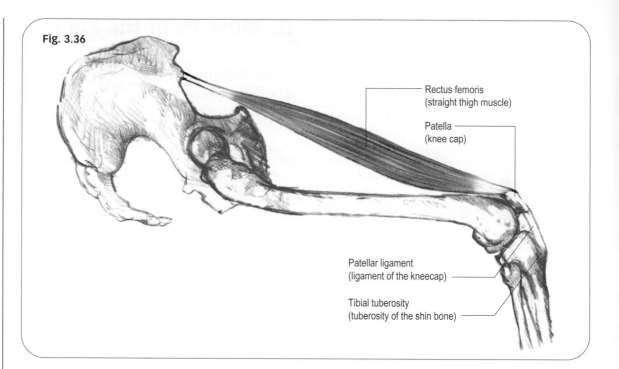

Fig. 3.36

Rectus femoris
(straight thigh muscle)

Patella
(knee cap)

Patellar ligament
(ligament of the kneecap)

Tibial tuberosity
(tuberosity of the shin bone)

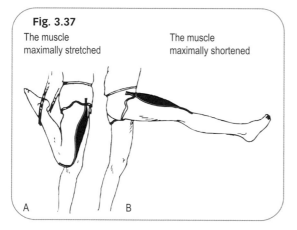

Fig. 3.37
The muscle
maximally stretched

The muscle
maximally shortened

A   B

the same collagen sheet as the vastus intermedius. The rest of the cells go straight to the outer and inner sides of the patella.

C. The rectus femoris starts on the spina iliaca anterior inferior (anterior inferior iliac spine) and passes in front of the vastus intermedius. The cells reach via a thick broad tendon down to the upper part of the patella.

The whole muscle group is called the quadriceps femoris (four-headed thigh muscle) (or 'quadriceps' for short) and all four individual components are in contact with the patella. This in turn is embedded in a thick tendon which inserts high up on the tibia at the tibial tuberosity.

Function:
Straighten the knee when working concentrically. Impede flexing of the knee joint when working eccentrically.

Their action is to straighten the knee and to stabilize and guide the patella so that it correctly glides in the depression formed by the femoral condyles (p. 53).

The main function of the patella is to enable the force exerted by the quadriceps to be redirected around the knee. At the same time it increases the leverage of the muscle. The thickness of the patella and its cartilage layer (~2 cm) lifts the tendon away from the centre of rotation of the knee joint (Figure 3.39). The force (F) from the muscle contraction gets a longer lever (l) to the centre of the movement. This makes the muscle effectively stronger because its effective strength is equal to the moment of force or torque ($F \times l$). With the patella, l (and thereby torque) will be ~25% larger than without.

The exercises shown in Figure 3.40 use the quadriceps femoris.

Fig. 3.38

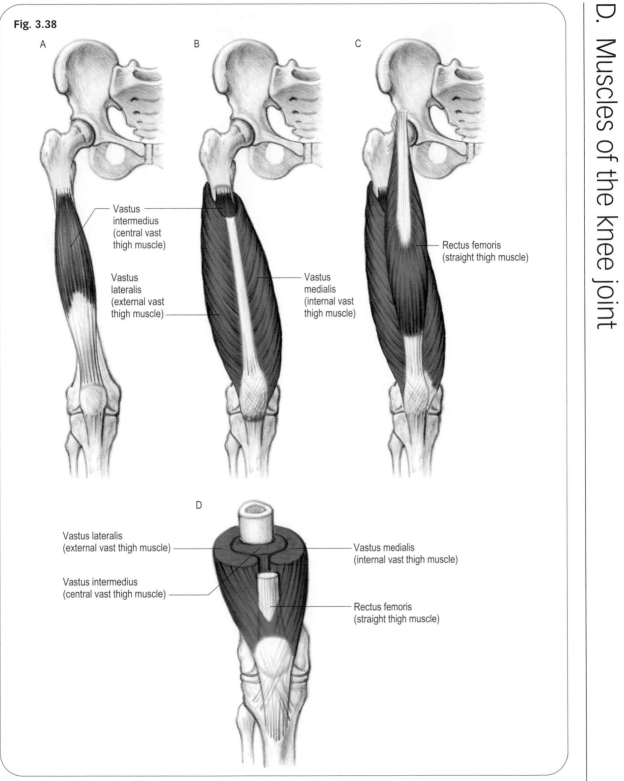

A

Vastus intermedius (central vast thigh muscle)

Vastus lateralis (external vast thigh muscle)

B

Vastus medialis (internal vast thigh muscle)

C

Rectus femoris (straight thigh muscle)

D

Vastus lateralis (external vast thigh muscle)

Vastus intermedius (central vast thigh muscle)

Vastus medialis (internal vast thigh muscle)

Rectus femoris (straight thigh muscle)

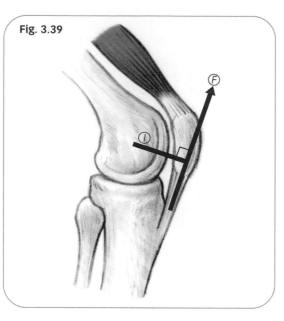

Fig. 3.39

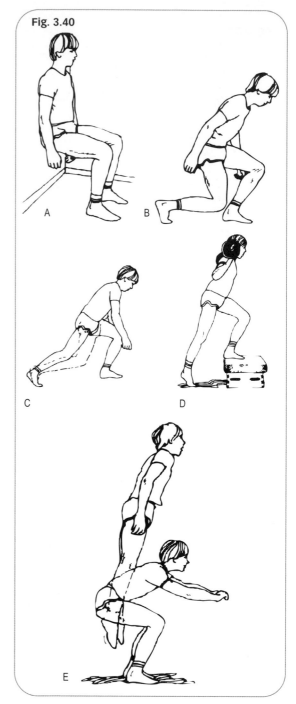

Fig. 3.40

Figure 3.40A. Sit with your back against a wall with a 90° angle between your hip and knee joints. The muscle acts statically.

Figure 3.40B. Stand with your weight on your left foot and place your right knee directly behind the tendon of your left heel. You will notice a distinct difference if you stand completely still in this position (static stress), or if you bounce lightly up and down (short periods of relaxation allow the blood to be supplied to the muscle).

Figure 3.40C. Start walking with long strides, each followed by an elastic stretch. Your bodyweight should be placed far forward over your leading foot. The halting movement trains the muscle eccentrically.

Figure 3.40D. Step up and down from a bench or part of a vaulting horse and – if your back is sufficiently strong – you could even carry a load on your shoulders. This exercise provides dynamic (mostly concentric) training.

Figure 3.40E. Jump up (concentric work) and down (eccentric work) on the spot. You must halt the movement before bending your knees too much (not more than a 90° angle at the knee joint, see Figures 3.41 and 3.42).

The work load in exercises A–E is greatest when the knee is flexed. The deeper you descend, the greater the work load will be. The muscles are subjected to large but harmless stress. However, the cartilage at the back of your patella will be subjected to harmful stress if you bend your knees too much. An explanation follows. (See Fig. 2.21 for diagrams and descriptions of how the origin and insertion of muscles are affected by muscle forces.)

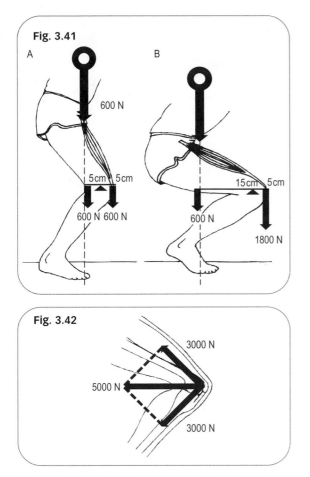

Fig. 3.41

A

600 N

5cm 5cm

600 N 600 N

B

15cm 5cm

600 N

1800 N

Fig. 3.42

3000 N

5000 N

3000 N

Examples of stress produced in the knee joint

Figure 3.41A. When standing on one leg (with slightly bent knee and centre of gravity 5 cm behind the axis of motion of the knee joint), the knee extensors, quadriceps femoris (four-headed thigh muscle) must contract with enough force to keep the body from collapsing and sitting down. According to the seesaw principle, the force of the muscle must equal that of gravity if the muscle's lever arm is also 5 cm.

Figure 3.41B. If the knee is flexed at a lesser angle than in (A), the distance between the vertical line and the axis of motion of the knee will become 15 cm, although the muscle's lever arm will remain unchanged at 5 cm. In example (B) the muscle force must be 3 × 600 N because its lever arm is three times less than that of the gravitational force.

With extreme bending of the knee a muscle force of 4–5 times the force of gravity

(bodyweight) may be required. The force that pulls the patella (kneecap) over the femur (thigh bone) can thus amount to 3000 N. Consequently, the patella is subjected to forces that together press it against the femur with a force that, at small angles, is almost double, i.e. 5000 N according to Figure 3.42. If exercises of this type are repeated frequently, the athlete runs a great risk of tearing the cartilage. The rule of thumb, never bend too deeply at the knees while they are subjected to stress (in the form of extra weights, speed, short stopping distance, etc.), is really worth following!

The calculations above show that the stress to which a straight knee is subjected is almost zero. Conversely, the deeper you bend, the greater the stress will become.

With the help of EMG (electromyography = the recording of muscle activity), it has been shown that the vastus medialis (internal vast thigh muscle) is most active during the final extension of the leg. In order to train this part of the quadriceps, it is necessary to construct exercises that put the greatest stress on the leg when the knee is fully extended. None of the exercises described in Figure 3.40 are of this type.

In the following exercises (Figure 3.43) the extended knee is subjected to intense loads (force to overcome).

In all three exercises the load is greatest when the knee is fully extended (the knee remains extended for static stress). These exercises particularly strengthen the vastus medialis, a muscle that is especially important for the stability of the knee. The femur and the tibia (shin bone) form a certain angle with each other. The patella is acted upon primarily along the direction of the thigh (rectus femoris (straight thigh muscle) and the vastus medialis and lateralis (internal and external vast thigh muscles)), i.e. slightly laterally, but the depression in which the patella glides, lies on a vertical line (Figure 3.44; anterior view).

The muscle whose job it is to guide the patella correctly, so that it is not drawn outwards and so that it does not 'scrape' against the lateral femoral condyle (external condyle of the thigh bone), is the vastus medialis. Its direction of pull is shown by the arrow F_m in Figure 3.44. This

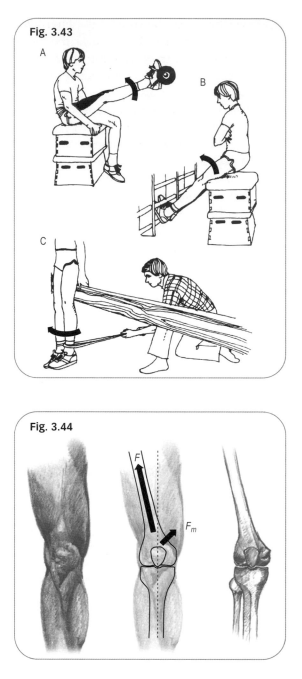

Fig. 3.43

Fig. 3.44

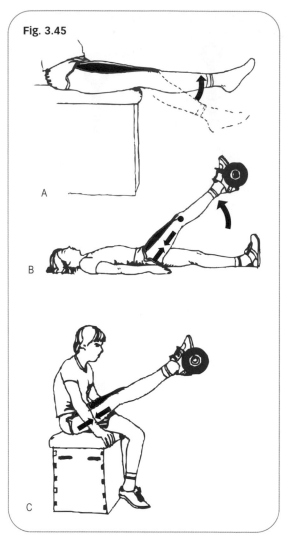

Fig. 3.45

Figure 3.45A. The quadriceps femoris muscle must overcome the weight of the lower leg. Its work load can be increased by placing a sandbag on the foot or wearing a weighted shoe.

Figure 3.45B. If the leg is lifted while straight, the weight of the lower leg still subjects the quadriceps femoris to stress. This exercise is more demanding than (A) because the muscles at the back of the thigh stretch and strive to flex the knee joint. Thus, the extensor (the quadriceps) has to work harder than in example (A).

Figure 3.45C. When a body sits, the pelvis tips forwards, which does not happen if it lies as shown in example (B). This causes the muscles at the back of the thigh to stretch even further. Thus, exercise (C) is heavier than exercise (B). Furthermore, it also subjects the flexors of the hip to stress.

muscle is weakened extremely quickly when the knee is injured. For this reason, a special training programme in which the extended knee is subjected to stress should be given top priority after the knee has been in a cast for a time. The diagrams in Figure 3.45A–C illustrate some relatively easy exercises that are aimed at building up strength after an accident. Their goal is to place the greatest load on the extended knee.

A well-trained elite high jumper, for example, could aim at being able to sit and lift a straight leg 45° above the horizontal plane with a load of 15 kg on his foot.

Knee flexors

When judging the value of different exercises designed for the knee extensors, one must take account of the antagonist muscles concerned, i.e. those situated at the back of the thigh. The collective name for these muscles is the hamstrings. They originate from the ischium (the lowermost part of the hip bone) and run towards the knee. There are three in all as shown in Figure 3.46A which is a view of the pelvis and femur (thigh bone) from behind. All three originate from the ischial tuberosity. The biceps femoris (two-headed thigh muscle) is inserted into the head of the fibula (calf bone). It can rotate the lower leg so that the foot points outwards. In Figure 3.46 you see the semimembranosus

muscle only on the left side and semitendinosus only on the right side. The reason is that the semitendinosus almost overlaps the semimembranosus so that the latter can hardly be seen beneath it. Of course all three muscles (these two and biceps femoris) exist in both legs.

Figure 3.47A and B respectively show the biceps femoris maximally contracted and maximally stretched. The semitendinosus and semimembranosus muscles are inserted into the medial tibial condyle (internal condyle of the shin bone); therefore they can rotate the lower leg inwards.

This group of muscles is called the hamstrings because their tendons can easily be felt at the back of the thigh. The distance between the origin and insertion of these hip extensors and knee flexors varies greatly depending upon the angle of the hip and knee joints.

In Figure 3.48 you see the relative positions and areas in the middle part of the thigh.

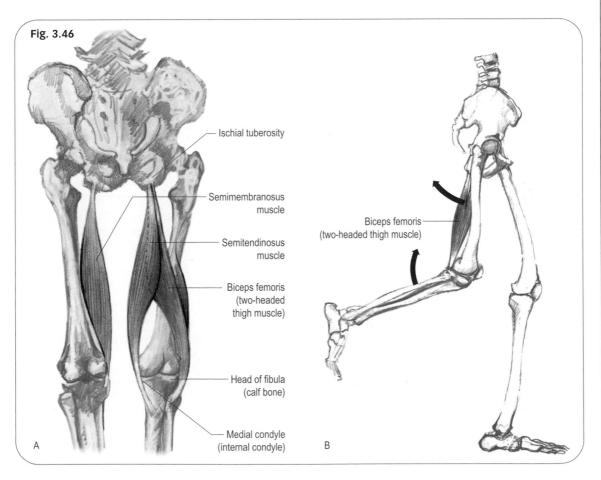

Fig. 3.46

Ischial tuberosity

Semimembranosus muscle

Semitendinosus muscle

Biceps femoris (two-headed thigh muscle)

Head of fibula (calf bone)

Medial condyle (internal condyle)

A

Biceps femoris (two-headed thigh muscle)

B

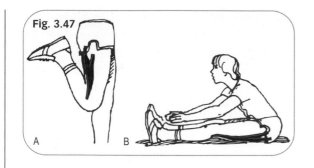

Fig. 3.47

A   B

Shortened muscles at the back of the thigh result in a stationary hip. When a person is unable to tip his pelvis forwards, he tries to compensate for this by bending forwards at his lumbar spine. Back trouble often results from the hamstrings being too short.

Flexibility exercises for the knee flexors

The following diagrams (Figure 3.49A–C) demonstrate stretching exercises for the knee flexors using the PNF (proprioceptive neuromuscular facilitation) method (p. 32).

Figure 3.49A. Assume this position without bending forwards at your lumbar spine, and keep your back straight. Tip your pelvis as far forwards as your thigh muscles will allow.

Figure 3.49B. Stand with your knees bent and your hands touching the ground. Then stretch your knees until you feel a comfortable tension at the back of your thigh. By supporting your hands on the ground you are taking the load off your back. If you straighten one leg at a time, the lifted leg will further unload your back. This exercise is best suited for those who already have relatively long hamstrings.

Figure 3.49C. Lie on your back and pull one leg – held straight – towards your chest.

Strength-developing exercises for the knee flexors

The exercises below (Figure 3.50A–D) are examples of different strength-developing exercises for the back of the thigh.

Figure 3.50A. A friend (or weighted shoe or rubber hose) should provide just enough resistance to allow you to change your knee angle with even movements. The resistance should not be so great that you are forced to bend at the hip in order to perform the movements. Moving in direction *a* means concentric work, direction *b* means eccentric work (see Figure 3.50B).

Figure 3.50B. By bending at the hip using the iliopsoas (i.e. tip your pelvis forwards), the origin of the hamstrings (the ischial tuberosity) will move further away from your lower leg. Thus, you stretch your flexors and thereby increase their strength (p. 17). This means that you subject your lumbar spine to stress in an unfavourable position, and this could lead to pain. Thus, you ought to press your hip down

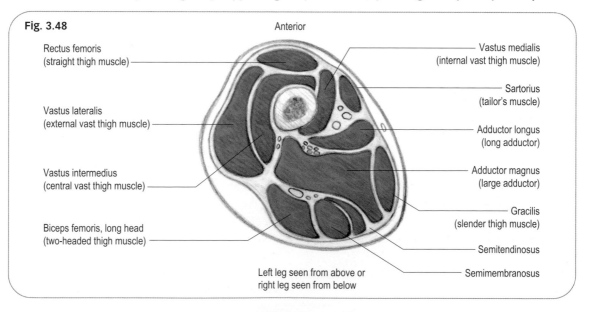

Fig. 3.48

Anterior

Rectus femoris (straight thigh muscle)

Vastus lateralis (external vast thigh muscle)

Vastus intermedius (central vast thigh muscle)

Biceps femoris, long head (two-headed thigh muscle)

Vastus medialis (internal vast thigh muscle)

Sartorius (tailor's muscle)

Adductor longus (long adductor)

Adductor magnus (large adductor)

Gracilis (slender thigh muscle)

Semitendinosus

Semimembranosus

Left leg seen from above or right leg seen from below

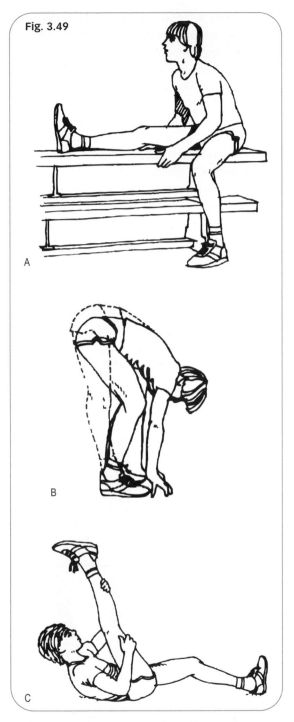

Fig. 3.49

A

B

C

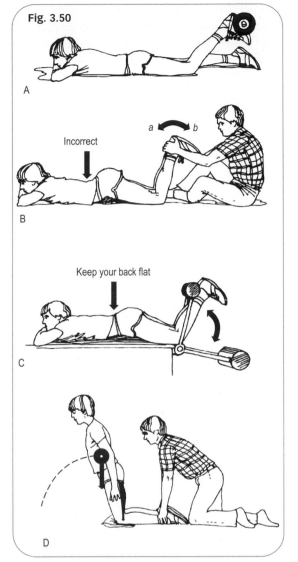

Fig. 3.50

A

Incorrect

a ⌒ *b*

B

Keep your back flat

C

D

and not strain it more than is necessary to perform the movement with your hips touching the ground.

Figure 3.50C. The same strength-developing apparatus that was used to train the knee extensors can be used to train the knee flexors, but keep your back flat.

Figure 3.50D. The following exercise is demanding. Kneel on a soft surface with your lower legs fixed. Then let your upper body fall slowly forwards and thereafter pull it back. Keep your hips straight. It is advisable to begin with small movements. This exercise subjects the muscles to great stress and can easily lead to a tendency for cramps if one is untrained. Here, it is the body's own weight that subjects the muscles to stress. The further the body's centre of gravity is placed in front of the knee joint, the greater is the moment of force the knee flexors must cancel. When the trunk is lowered, the muscles act eccentrically; when it is raised to the vertical position they are acting concentrically.

In order to train the muscles at the back of the thigh for coordination and speed you can run with short quick strides; sprint and try to kick your buttocks; or cycle quickly (in first gear).

E. Lower leg and foot

A muscle group that is very important for jumping and running is the triceps surae (three-headed calf muscle) (Figure 3.51A and B). This muscle has three parts: the gastrocnemius (twin calf muscle) with its two heads of origin (one from each of the femoral condyles (condyles of the thigh bone), and the soleus (flounder muscle) (a flat muscle originating from the back of the lower leg). Together these three parts converge into the Achilles tendon (heel tendon), which is inserted into the calcaneus (heel bone) (Figure 3.51C).

The gastrocnemius bends (or flexes) both the knee and the ankle so that the body can be raised on its toes (plantarflexion). The soleus muscle acts only on the ankle joint.

Figure 3.51D. Place the balls of your feet against something that will raise them 5 cm above your heels. Stand on your toes, and then

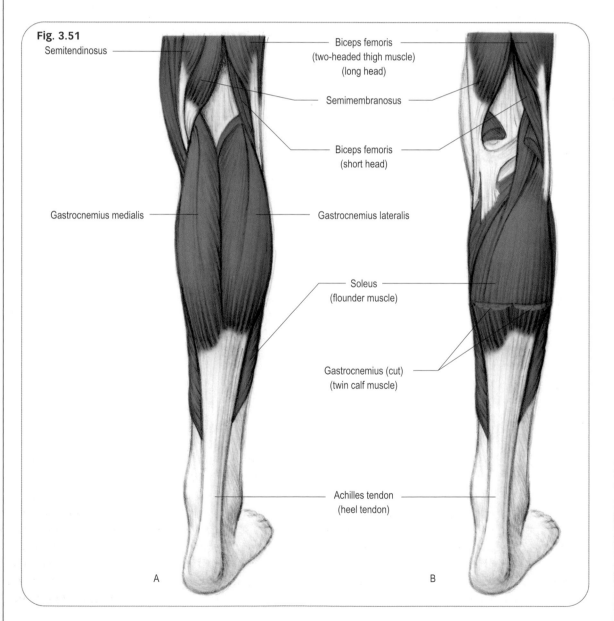

Fig. 3.51

Semitendinosus

Biceps femoris
(two-headed thigh muscle)
(long head)

Semimembranosus

Biceps femoris
(short head)

Gastrocnemius medialis

Gastrocnemius lateralis

Soleus
(flounder muscle)

Gastrocnemius (cut)
(twin calf muscle)

Achilles tendon
(heel tendon)

A

B

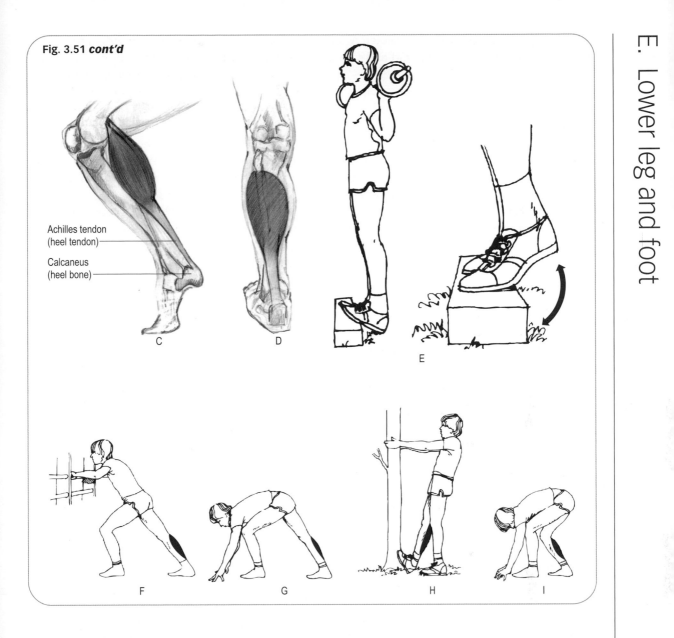

Fig. 3.51 *cont'd*

Achilles tendon
(heel tendon)

Calcaneus
(heel bone)

C

D

E

F

G

H

I

return to your original position (Fig. 3.51E). This exercise can be done quickly many times (dynamic endurance) or with a heavy weight five or six times (maximal strength training) (p. 37). When pressing upwards the muscles are trained concentrically and when descending they are trained eccentrically. For a very short period – when the heel is in contact with the ground – the muscle can relax in its extended position. This has a certain stretching effect.

If you want to stretch your gastrocnemius you can do the following exercise. Stand against a wall (Figure 3.51F) or bent forward (G) with support for your hands. Then, move one leg as far as possible behind you keeping your heel on the ground.

The muscle can be activated with the PNF (proprioceptive neuromuscular facilitation) method by pressing the ball of your foot against the ground for a few seconds. Another good way is to plant the ball of your foot against a tree and pull yourself carefully forwards with your arms so that the calf muscles are stretched (Figure 3.47H). If your knees are straight, then you will be stretching only your gastrocnemius, (F), (G) and (H). If your knees are bent, the soleus is stretched (I). The latter is often neglected. When it is, the calf muscle will still feel stiff and sore.

The foot

When the calf muscle is too short, the foot tends to assume a position with downward-pointing toes (Figure 3.52). The muscles that hold the foot up (situated at the front of the lower leg between the tibia (shin bone) and fibula (calf bone), see p. 76), are thus forced to work constantly with raised tension (tone) in order to hold the foot in its normal position. Such tension may lie behind the pain that is experienced in the lower leg when an athlete trains too much in one session, or runs on hard surfaces, etc.

When we take a closer look at how the heel tendon is attached to the calcaneus (heel bone), we can easily understand how mechanically correctly the muscles of the body are arranged. If the Achilles tendon (heel tendon) were attached as shown in Figure 3.53A its lever arm (i.e. ability to turn the ankle) would have less and less

effect the more the body is raised on the toes (l_1 would be reduced to l_2).

However, the Achilles tendon is attached to the calcaneus near its base (Figure 3.53B), which means that the lever arm (l) remains about the same length regardless of whether the whole foot is firmly planted on the ground or whether the body is standing on its toes.

Figure 3.54 (lateral view) shows that the tendon is protected from scraping against the calcaneus by a bursa that is situated between the tendon and the bone.

Movements of the foot

The foot can move round two axes (Figure 3.55). The movements around axis I are called flexion and extension. Movements around axis 2 are called pronation and supination.

Skeleton of the foot

The skeleton of the foot is divided into tarsals (bones of the ankle), metatarsals (bones of the foot) and phalanges (bones of the toes) (Figure 3.56).

Extension and flexion take place between the talus (the ankle bone) and the tibia (shin bone) and fibula (calf bone). The joint involved is called the ankle joint.

Supination and pronation take place between the talus and the navicular bone ('boat-shaped'

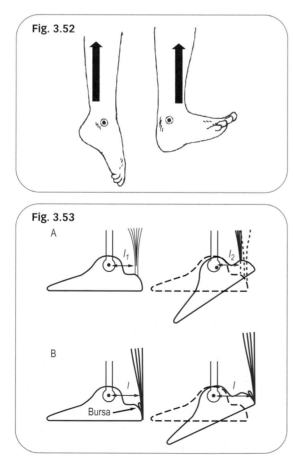

Fig. 3.52

Fig. 3.53

A

B

Bursa

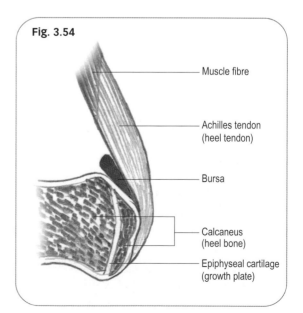

Fig. 3.54

Muscle fibre

Achilles tendon (heel tendon)

Bursa

Calcaneus (heel bone)

Epiphyseal cartilage (growth plate)

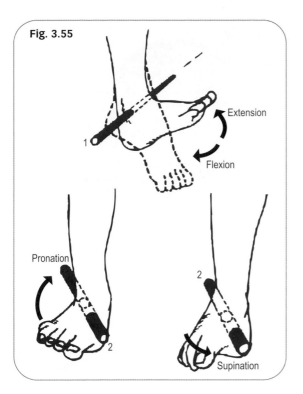

Fig. 3.55

1

Extension

Flexion

Pronation

2

2

Supination

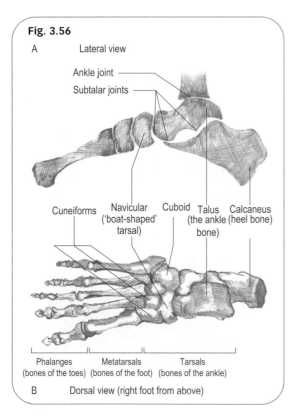

Fig. 3.56

A   Lateral view

Ankle joint

Subtalar joints

Cuneiforms

Navicular ('boat-shaped' tarsal)

Cuboid

Talus (the ankle bone)

Calcaneus (heel bone)

Phalanges (bones of the toes)

Metatarsals (bones of the foot)

Tarsals (bones of the ankle)

B   Dorsal view (right foot from above)

tarsal) and the calcaneus (heel bone). The joint involved is known as the subtalar joint.

Supination and pronation take place simultaneously between several articulating surfaces that together form the subtalar joints.

Movements of the ankle and subtalar joints are independent of each other. The movements of the foot at these joints are controlled, as usual, by the muscles. If the muscles are unable to prevent movements that are too great or too sudden, the joint is still protected by the ligaments of the foot.

The ankle ligaments arise from the prominent lower ends (the malleoli) of the tibia and fibula and spread out down towards the articulating ankle bones. Thus, the medial (internal) ligament of the ankle arises from the medial malleolus of the tibia and is inserted into the calcaneus, talus and navicular bones. It is called the deltoid ligament.

There are three separate ligaments making up the lateral (external) ligament. They all arise from the lateral malleolus of the fibula. One of them extends forwards and is inserted into the talus, one passes downwards to be attached to the calcaneus, and the third one extends backwards towards the back part of the talus. Figure 3.57A shows the medial ligament otherwise known as the deltoid ligament; Figure 3.57B shows the lateral ligaments.

The origin of the deltoid ligament corresponds to the axis of motion of the ankle joint. Thus it is always taut. The origin of the lateral ligament is situated below the axis of motion. Hence, its posterior part is taut when the foot points upwards and the anterior part is taut when the ankle is stretched. When injured, the ligament either suffers a partial rupture or is completely torn. In many cases the ligament remains intact but the malleolus is broken off.

Muscles of the foot

The most important flexor (see p. 72) is the triceps surae (three-headed calf muscle). It is, however, assisted by other muscles whose tendons can be felt and seen behind the malleoli. The most important extensors (1, 2, 3, in Figure 3.58) are found at the front of the leg between the tibia (shin bone) and fibula (calf bone). Their tendons

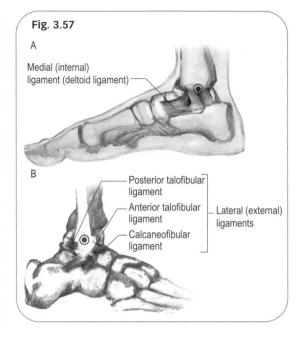

Fig. 3.57

A

Medial (internal) ligament (deltoid ligament)

B

Posterior talofibular ligament

Anterior talofibular ligament — Lateral (external) ligaments

Calcaneofibular ligament

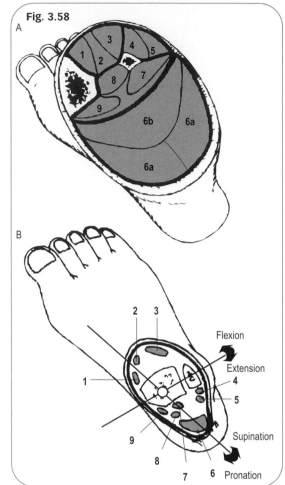

Fig. 3.58

A

6b   6a

6a

B

2   3

Flexion

Extension

1   4

5

9

Supination

8

7   6   Pronation

can easily be felt on the top of the foot at the base of the tibia. Pronation is brought about by the two muscles whose tendons can be felt beneath the lateral (external) malleolus of the tibia (4, 5). Supination is produced mainly by the three muscles whose tendons pass behind and beneath the medial (internal) malleolus of the tibia (7, 8, 9). Figure 3.58B shows their locations in relation to the different axes of motion.

Figure 3.58A is a view from above, half-way up the tibia, Figure 3.58B is a view at the level of the ankle joint.

The numbers in the diagrams refer to the following muscles.

1. Tibialis anterior (anterior shin bone muscle).
2. Extensor hallucis longus (long big toe extensor).
3. Extensor digitorum longus (long toe extensor).
4. Peroneus longus (long calf muscle).
5. Peroneus brevis (short calf muscle).
6. Triceps surae (three-headed calf muscle) (6a gastrocnemius; 6b soleus).
7. Flexor hallucis longus (long big toe flexor).
8. Flexor digitorum longus (long toe flexor).
9. Tibialis posterior (posterior shin bone muscle).

Figure 3.58 has arrows showing how the foot moves in flexion–extension and in supination–pronation. For example, flexion will happen if any of the muscles 4–9 contract and move the heel upwards ➤. Contractions in 4–5 will produce pronation ➤.

When describing the structure and function of the foot it is useful to review the concept of 'arches'. There are three types (Figure 3.59, medial view):

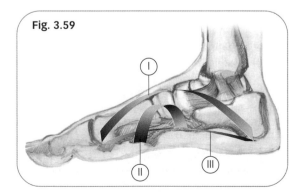

Fig. 3.59

I

II   III

1. Movement arch
2. Support arch
3. Anterior arch

Running subjects the support arch to stress. Notice how a running shoe wears down at the outer border of the heel and under the big toe. The other arches – which are supported by *ligaments*, the *wedge-shaped construction of the bones* and the *muscles* – give the foot its elasticity. Departures from the normal appearance can either lead to an arch that is too high (not very common) or too low (flatfoot). The latter may be due to the ligament being stretched which, in turn, could be the result of subjecting the foot to severe stress (running on hard surfaces without arch support) or imbalance of muscle strength between the different muscles. The structures that affect the movement arch are listed below (Figure 3.60). The structures marked with a plus sign have a tendency to raise the movement arch and those marked with a minus sign tend to lower it.

The most common foot injuries are those sustained by the lateral ligament of the ankle joint. These injuries are caused by lopsided gait. The majority of injuries can be avoided by wearing appropriate shoes. Shoes that are worn down on one side only (on the outside of the heel) are usually the culprit. Another common cause of foot injury is a surface that provides so much friction that the shoes stick at the slightest contact. The muscles that pronate (i.e. lift the outer border with the result that a shoe does not become firmly fixed on the ground too soon) are the peroneus longus and brevis (numbered 4, 5 in Figure 3.58). It is very important that these muscles are strong

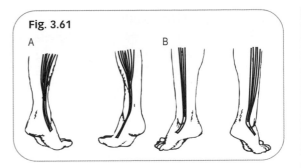

Fig. 3.61

A   B

and can react quickly. The calf muscles and their agonists can be trained with 'toe push-ups'.

If you stand on your toes with the sole of your foot pointing inwards as shown below (Figure 3.61A) and push up balancing on the outside of your foot, you will be engaging 7, 8 and 9 (see Figure 3.58). If you stand on your toes with the sole pointing outwards (Figure 3.61B), 4 and 5 (Figure 3.58) will be engaged. Coordination and speed can be developed by standing and balancing on an unstable object.

You can both control and develop your ability to finely adjust your foot position in the following way: stand on one leg with a bent knee, keeping your arms by your sides and eyes shut. It is always considerably more difficult to balance on one leg if that leg has recently been injured, as it takes time to retrain fine motor ability (Figure 3.62). The risk of new sprains is obvious if rehabilitation is not hastened.

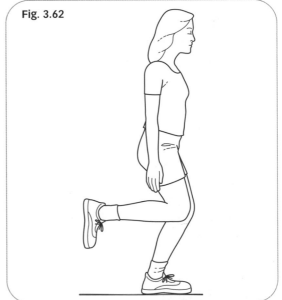

Fig. 3.62

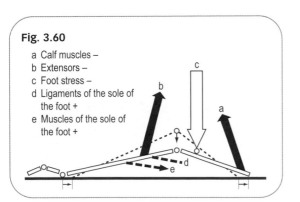

Fig. 3.60

a Calf muscles –
b Extensors –
c Foot stress –
d Ligaments of the sole of
  the foot +
e Muscles of the sole of
  the foot +

Periostitis ('shin splints')

A problem facing many athletes is inflammation of the periosteum (the membrane covering the bones), i.e. periostitis. The muscles responsible for lifting the foot (1, 2, 3 (see Figure 3.58)) are situated at the front of the leg between the tibia (shin bone) and fibula (calf bone). They are enclosed in a fascia (tough connective tissue). The interosseous membrane between the tibia and fibula serves as a direct point of origin for some parts of the muscles. The rest of the muscles grow directly out of the bone walls and pass through the periosteum, which has intimate contact with the fascia.

The periosteum may become detached from the bone due to the force of the muscle contraction or high tension in the muscle fascia, which is inserted into the bone through the periosteum. Small haemorrhages and inflammations appear in the microscopic cavities that form between the detached periosteum and the bone.

As mentioned earlier, athletes who train by running a great deal often sustain periostitis. The healing process will be delayed if they continue to run, as by doing so the worn tissues are not given time to heal. Pain can also be caused by changing the running surface or suddenly increasing the amount of training. The muscles – which are confined within the muscle fascia – swell (fill with blood) more than the fascia will permit. The pressure that then builds up leads to a pain resembling periostitis pain. Such increased pressure in a muscle compartment is referred to as 'closed compartment syndrome'.

A successful surgical method for treating severe cases of increased pressure is to cleave the muscle fascia by making a longitudinal slit between the tibia and fibula on the fore side of the leg. In this way the pressure in the anterior muscle compartment will be reduced.

Running on hard surfaces can lead to a complaint similar to periostitis. The sudden and excessive stresses to which the leg is subjected at each stride can, at worst, give rise to microscopic small splits in the outer lamella (layer) of the bone. This type of complaint heals with greater difficulty than the more common periostitis.

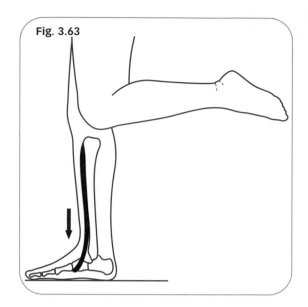

Fig. 3.63

The wearing of unsuitable shoes when running on hard surfaces causes the movement arch to fall at each stride. The tibialis anterior (anterior shin bone muscle) (numbered 1 in Figure 3.58), which is attached to the arch (see Figure 3.63), will fall and thus pull on its origin with a great deal of force. This is especially the case when the whole foot is planted on the ground instead of the heel striking first. The shoe should be built up at the arch to give it support.

F. Strengthening the legs

When training muscles that pass the hip joint you should consider the fact that the joint can move around three axes. That means movements in six different directions: extension–flexion, abduction–adduction and outward–inward rotation. The most common training apparatus and choice of exercises usually engage the first four of these directions. The muscles are not trained as individuals but as groups of muscles where all contribute to handling the stress they are exposed to. Yet there is always some muscle which is strongest and that's the one usually mentioned when you discuss a specific movement.

If the strength of a muscle group is different in different parts of the movement, it is important to know about its strength profile (see for example Figure 2.26). When the differences are great its useful to split up the exercise. Train the weaker part with low weights and maybe a somewhat different pattern of movement than the stronger part.

From here on you can read about muscle groups in much the same order of appearance as the individual muscles earlier in this chapter.

Hip extension

- **Gluteus maximus** (large buttock muscle)
- Gluteus medius (intermediate buttock muscle)
- Gluteus minimus (small buttock muscle)
- **Hamstrings**
- Adductor magnus (large adductor muscle)

This muscle group is trained when you go from a standing position to a squat and back again. The load you have to control depends on how much you weigh 'above' your hip joint (about 65% of your body weight according to Figure 6.65). In this exercise you are also flexing your knees, which automatically stresses the knee extensors,

the quadriceps femoris (four-headed thigh muscle). The deeper you bend the greater the stress. That does not mean that you all of a sudden get heavier; it happens because both the hip joint and the knee joint move further and further out from the line of action of gravity the deeper you go (Figures 3.64 and 3.65). The moment of force around the joints thus becomes greater and the muscles have to produce more force to cope (Fig. 3.41). At the end of the downward motion you brake your speed with your hip and knee extensors working eccentrically. On the way up they work concentrically. If the force then is high enough you will jump up from the floor. That is a way to stress the muscles to near maximum. The load for this exercise can be increased by:

- A handle weight or a disc bar on your shoulders.
- Deeper positions when turning up again. (But avoid bending the knee to less than 90°.)
- Higher speed of movement. (Be sure to have control before reaching the lowest point.)

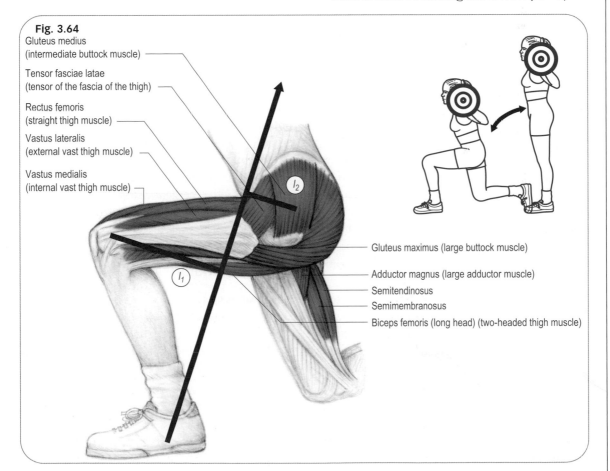

Fig. 3.64

Gluteus medius (intermediate buttock muscle)

Tensor fasciae latae (tensor of the fascia of the thigh)

Rectus femoris (straight thigh muscle)

Vastus lateralis (external vast thigh muscle)

Vastus medialis (internal vast thigh muscle)

l_2

l_1

Gluteus maximus (large buttock muscle)

Adductor magnus (large adductor muscle)

Semitendinosus

Semimembranosus

Biceps femoris (long head) (two-headed thigh muscle)

Fig. 3.65

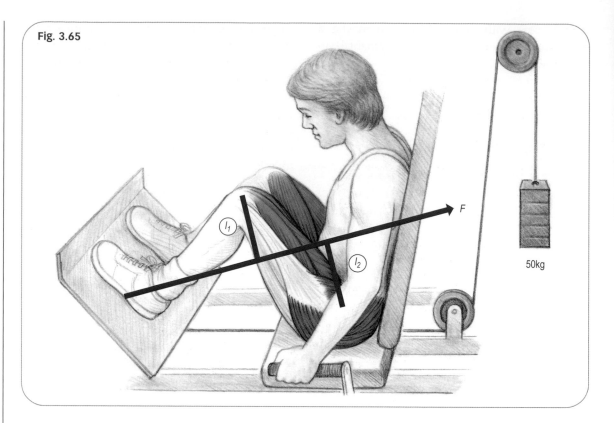

If you weigh 70 kg, the load on your hips is ~ 50 kg). The load can now be raised by 10% at a time by choosing handles or a disc bar where you repeatedly add 5 kg. With a 50 kg disc bar you have doubled the weight on your muscles. Note that you can easily achieve the same thing by doing squats on one leg with your body weight as the only load. If you choose this option you must be careful with balance (use your hands as a support and be ready to use your other leg if needed). Don't do deep or fast movements due to the high risk of accidents! If you choose to jump up from the floor (with or without extra load) you will also engage the calf muscle.

One of the most common forms of training apparatus for hip and knee extensors is some sort of chair where you 'half sit' and push a platform horizontally in front of you. You choose the load from a weight box. The construction makes the load press you against a squatting position. If no complicated devices multiply the weight by some unknown factor you can choose 50 kg in order to stress your muscles in the same way as standing up and doing squats with no extra loads. The advantage of the apparatus is the security arrangements that stop you from sinking too deep and so getting hurt. You will notice that muscles are stronger when breaking a movement (in this case going back) than when they try to push forwards (see p. 21). With too much weight you might be able to stop the movement but you are not strong enough to come up again. In an apparatus with emergency stop you can just 'step out' but with a disc bar on your shoulder an accident is close.

Knee extension

- **Quadriceps**
  - Vastus medialis (internal vast thigh muscle)
  - Vastus lateralis (external vast thigh muscle)
  - Vastus intermedius (central vast thigh muscle)
  - Rectus femoris (straight thigh muscle)
- Tensor fasciae latae (tensor of the fascia of the thigh) (via iliotibial tract)
- Gluteus maximus (large buttock muscle) (via iliotibial tract)

Both hip and knee extensors were used in the exercises discussed above. The weaker of the two groups decides what kind of load you can work with. Mostly it is the knee extensors that impose the limit. In order to strengthen the knee extensors you should use a chair that forces your knees to bend without influence on the hip joint. (Figure 3.66)

The knee extensors have a strength profile (described in Figure 2.26A) such that the muscles are strongest in the middle part of the movement when you are sitting in the chair. Most apparatus nowadays has unsymmetrical wheels so the force creates less torque at the beginning and end of the motion and more in the middle where the muscles are stronger.

If you want to train different individual components of the quadriceps femoris (four-headed thigh muscle) you should know that vastus medialis is more active the closer your knee is to straight. By contrast vastus lateralis is more active close to the deep bent position, as shown in Figures 3.67 and 3.68.

When we looked at hip extension we automatically had to take into account the associated knee extension. It is now logical to continue with knee flexion before returning to more hip exercises.

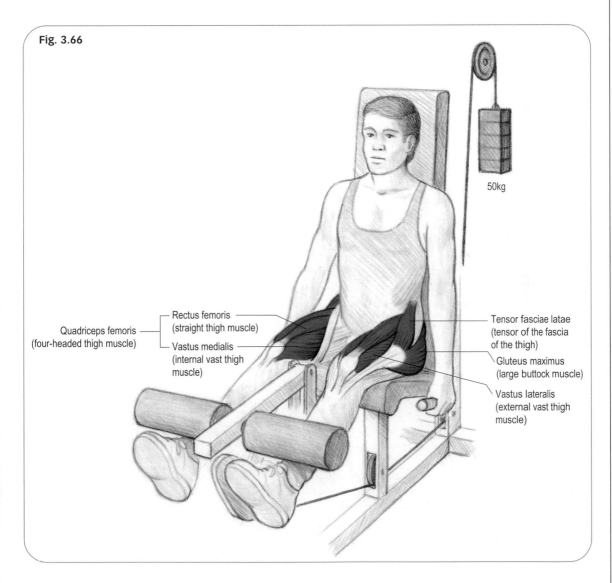

Fig. 3.66

50kg

Quadriceps femoris (four-headed thigh muscle)

Rectus femoris (straight thigh muscle)

Vastus medialis (internal vast thigh muscle)

Tensor fasciae latae (tensor of the fascia of the thigh)

Gluteus maximus (large buttock muscle)

Vastus lateralis (external vast thigh muscle)

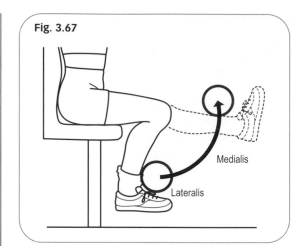

Fig. 3.67

Medialis

Lateralis

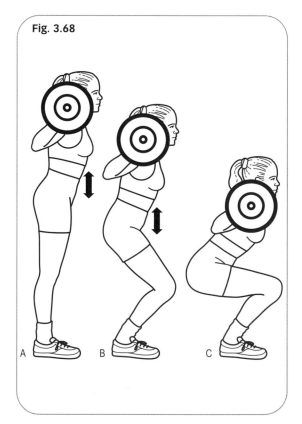

Fig. 3.68

A   B   C

Knee flexion

- **Hamstrings**
  - –Biceps femoris (two-headed thigh muscle)
  - –Semitendinosus
  - –Semimembranosus
- Gracilis (slender thigh muscle)
- Sartorius (tailor's muscle)
- Gastrocnemius (twin calf muscle)

The hamstrings are primarily knee flexors (but also hip extensors). They can be isolated and trained in apparatus where the hip is locked (Figure 3.69) and all movement takes place at the knees. Here it can be useful to look at the strength profile (Figure 3.70) and discuss what kind of influence it has on positions and loads when training. The muscle group is strongest when the hip is straight and the knee is slightly bent.

If you stand up and lift your lower leg (maybe with some extra load attached) from straight knee to a 90° bent position, the imposed torque will be in accord with Figure 3.70A. If you lie face down on a bench with 45° incline, the torque changes to the form shown in Figure 3.70B. If you lie on the floor the load is as in Figure 3.70C. The alternative that best adjusts to the knee flexors natural strength is Figure 3.70B.

Hamstrings work vigorously when you run fast. Their most important job is, immediately after the forefoot leaves the ground, rapidly to lift the heel towards the buttock. When the leg is completely bent it is much easier for the hip flexors to swing the leg forward fast. To be able to do this effectively it is important that the hamstrings are strongest in the position the leg is when the forefoot leaves the ground. It would be a waste if hamstrings were strongest at some other position. The muscles in the human leg are designed for standing upright and running fast on two legs. You train exactly correctly by doing natural things such as walking, running, jumping, lifting, pushing, pulling and carrying. Regardless of whether you do these activities freely or use specially designed apparatus you ought to have natural movement patterns as a guideline. This goes also for speed, load and movements.

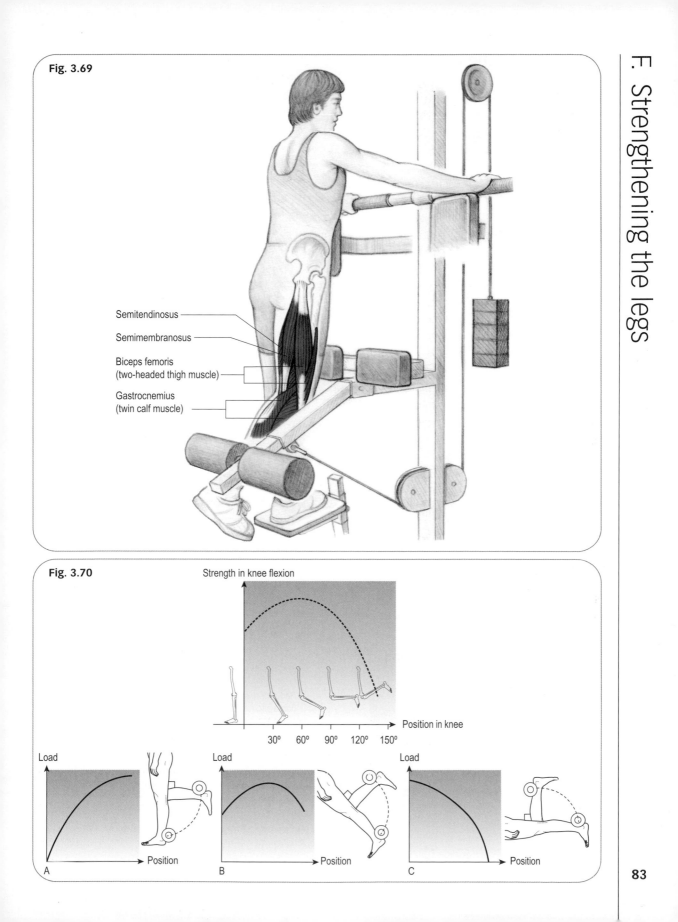

Fig. 3.69

Semitendinosus

Semimembranosus

Biceps femoris
(two-headed thigh muscle)

Gastrocnemius
(twin calf muscle)

Fig. 3.70

Strength in knee flexion

Position in knee

30°   60°   90°   120°   150°

Load

Position

A

Load

Position

B

Load

Position

C

Adduction in the hip joint

- **The groin muscles**
  - Adductor magnus (large adductor)
  - Adductor longus (long adductor)
  - Adductor brevis (short adductor)
  - Pectineus ('comb' muscle)
- Sartorius (tailor's muscle) (not shown in Figure 3.71)
- Gracilis (slender thigh muscle)
- Iliopsoas (not shown in Figure 3.71)

This big muscle group is very involved in handling the leg when we walk and run. If you look more closely at the adductors you realize that they can contribute to hip flexion as well as hip extension. Figure 3.72 shows how adductor longus is a flexor and adductor magnus is an extensor depending on their different origin. This means that, for example, adductor longus can help swinging the leg forward and adductor magnus decides when to stop and start dragging it backwards.

You train the whole group a little extra if you speed up and if you take longer strides than usual. Extra load can be achieved by rubber bands, pulling devices aimed straight or obliquely outwards. You let the leg be brought out, you break the movement and overcome the resistance and force the leg back to the starting position. You have to have good support, holding on to something stable, otherwise you expose the supporting leg to static (more tiring) load of the same magnitude as the moving leg you were supposed to exercise.

A very effective way of training all muscles in the leg is to make a number of jumps in different 'clock directions' (Figure 3.73). Imagine standing on both feet in the centre of a big clock. Start by jumping 4–5 times so your right foot lands on 12 o'clock and bounce back immediately landing on both feet in the centre. Another 4–5 jumps to 1 o'clock, 2 o'clock and so on always with your chest against 12. When you have made backward jumps to 6 o'clock still on the right leg you shift to the left leg and continue

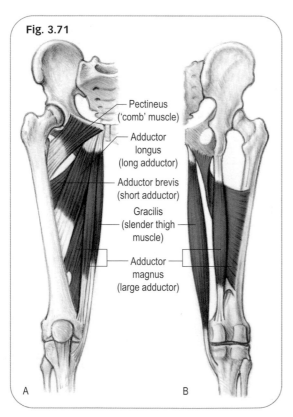

Fig. 3.71

Pectineus ('comb' muscle)

Adductor longus (long adductor)

Adductor brevis (short adductor)

Gracilis (slender thigh muscle)

Adductor magnus (large adductor)

A   B

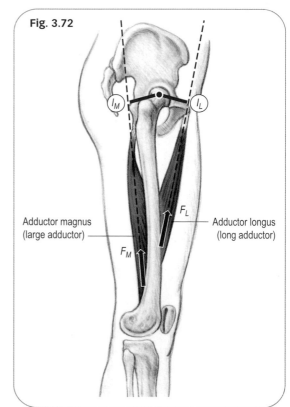

Fig. 3.72

I_M I_L

Adductor magnus (large adductor)

F_L

F_M

Adductor longus (long adductor)

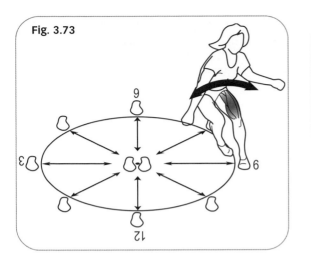

Fig. 3.73

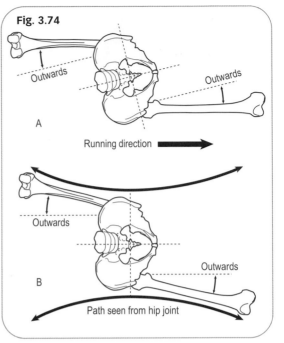

Fig. 3.74

Outwards

Outwards

A

Running direction ➡

Outwards

Outwards

B

Path seen from hip joint

through all directions 6–12. Good shoes, small jumps for the first sessions and no slippery floors are the essentials.

You could experiment with some sort of weight vest.

When you walk or run, the pelvis turns a couple of degrees (Fig. 3.74A). This causes the leg (even if it swings straight forward in the running direction) to move outwards a little at the hip joint. Seen from the pelvis the femur (thigh bone) moves in an elliptically shaped path (Figure 3.74B). No wonder we need so many and such strong muscles to be able to control ~15-kg legs moving in 'all' directions when running at full speed. Injured and over-used groin muscles are very hard to heal. It's almost impossible to rest them completely because they are used in every step we take. It's important for athletes to be strong and flexible in this group of muscles. When training, concentrate on medium load and many repetitions instead of heavy load and few reps.

Hip abduction

- Gluteus maximus (large buttock muscle)
- Gluteus minimus (small buttock muscle)
- Gluteus medius (intermediate buttock muscle)
- Sartorius (tailor's muscle)
- Tensor fasciae latae (tensor of the fascia of the thigh)

The three first are active when you land on one leg as you run or jump as in Figure 3.73. Running up a slope forces you to work hard concentrically. Running downhill with long strides trying to keep the speed low, is a tough way to eccentrically stress your abductors. Figure 3.75 shows one other way to train them. How to train the hip flexors will be dealt together with the abdominal muscles in the next chapter. The hip flexors and the abdominal muscles work closely together and are sometimes hard to individualize.

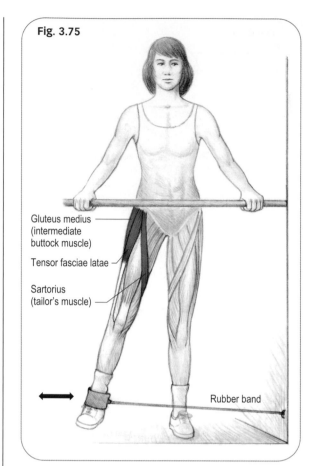

Fig. 3.75

Gluteus medius (intermediate buttock muscle)

Tensor fasciae latae

Sartorius (tailor's muscle)

Rubber band

Chapter 4

Anatomy and function of the trunk

Spinal column and vertebrae

The vertebral column consists of seven cervical (of the neck) vertebrae, which are numbered and usually written as C1, . . ., C7; 12 dorsal (or thoracic, i.e. of the chest) vertebrae T1, . . ., T12; and five lumbar vertebrae L1, . . ., L5 (Figure 4.1).

Between the vertebrae there are intervertebral discs made up of an outer ring of fibrocartilage (annulus fibrosus) and a more pulpy centre (nucleus pulposus) (Figure 4.2). Thus, the disc, with its tough fibrocartilage rim and soft, pulpy, highly elastic centre, acts as a shock absorber. Discs make up about one-third of the height of the vertebral column. Figures 4.3 and 4.4 respectively show vertebrae from above and from the side.

When two vertebrae are placed on top of each other (Figure 4.3) there is a substantial space between the stalks or pedicles of each vertebra; this is called the intervertebral foramen or opening. It is through this space that the nerves pass from the spinal cord (Figure 4.2) and reach out to all the different parts of the body.

The following characteristics of a vertebra can be distinguished in Figures 4.3 and 4.4 (top and side view respectively).

Body.
Neural arch.
Intervertebral foramen.
Transverse outgrowth or process.
Spinous outgrowth or process.
Articular outgrowth or process.

We are prevented from leaning too far back by the spinous processes and the tension of a long ligament that runs down the front of the spinal column (anterior longitudinal ligament) (Figure 4.5; side and top view respectively).

Forward bending is restricted partly by the back muscles, partly by the elastic ligament, which runs between the posterior parts of the neural arches (ligamentum flavum), and partly by the ligament that runs down the back of the vertebral bodies (i.e. in the anterior part of the intervertebral foramen). This latter ligament is called the posterior longitudinal ligament.

The back complaints of athletes are often due to the spine being subjected to excessive or uneven stress, or the body being subjected to sudden movements while it is in an unfavourable position.

The back complaints of non-athletes are often due to poorly trained back muscles (even poorly trained muscles of the legs and abdomen), the wear and tear of lifting objects in

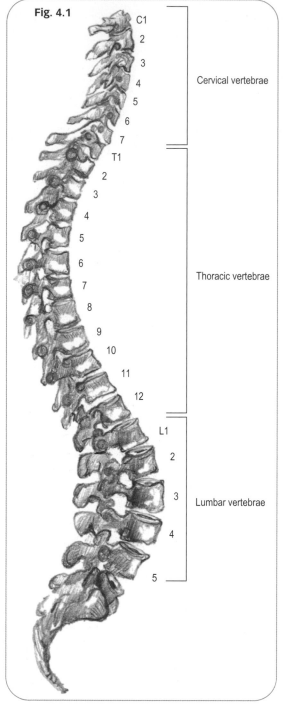

Fig. 4.1

C1
2
3
4
5
6
7

Cervical vertebrae

T1
2
3
4
5
6
7
8
9
10
11
12

Thoracic vertebrae

L1
2
3
4
5

Lumbar vertebrae

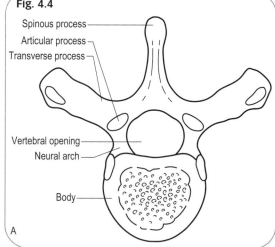

Fig. 4.2

Superior view

Spinal cord

Spinal nerve

Nucleus pulposus

Annulus fibrosus

Fig. 4.3

Annulus fibrosus
Nucleus pulposus

Intervertebral foramen

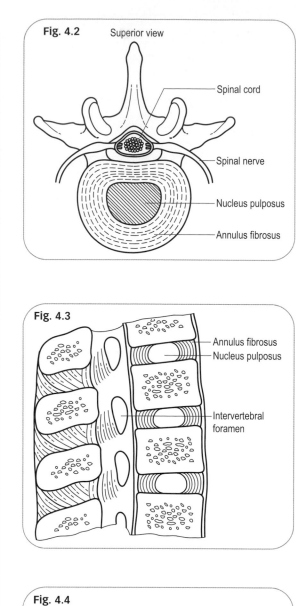

Fig. 4.4

Spinous process
Articular process
Transverse process

Vertebral opening
Neural arch

Body

A

a lopsided manner, sitting still or working in a position where the body is tilted forwards.

The pressure inside a disc varies according to the position of the body and external stress. The position that the body can assume, to ensure that the least amount of pressure is placed on the lumbar spine, is shown in Figure 4.6A. Thus, lie

Fig. 4.4

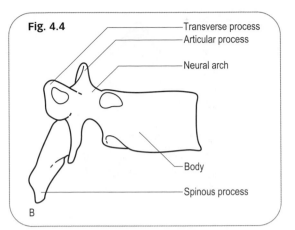

Transverse process
Articular process
Neural arch
Body
Spinous process

B

Fig. 4.6

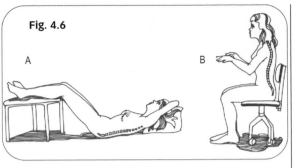

A

B

Fig. 4.5

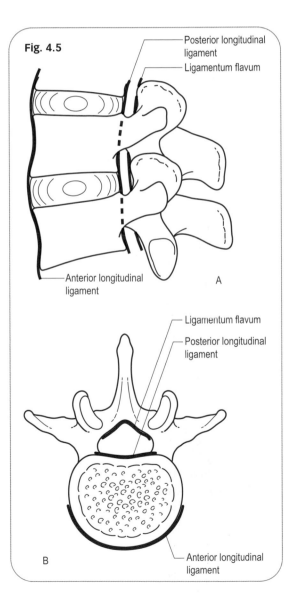

Posterior longitudinal ligament
Ligamentum flavum

Anterior longitudinal ligament

A

Ligamentum flavum
Posterior longitudinal ligament

Anterior longitudinal ligament

B

on your back and support your lower legs on, say, a chair so that the iliopsoas does not pull (and thereby increase disc pressure) on your spine. When a person is standing, as shown in Figure 4.7, a line from the centre of gravity (CG) to the ground (vertical midline) passes about 5 cm in front of the centre of disc L3, and the back muscles lie about 5 cm behind it. Hence, the muscle force must equal 400 N in order to prevent the upper body from falling forwards. The force acting on the disc is 400 + 400 = 800 N. Sitting positions produce greater disc pressure than standing positions, a fact that is unknown to many! As shown in Figure 4.8, when a person sits, the vertical midline passes about 15 cm in front of L3. The muscle's lever arm is 5 cm (as in standing). Therefore, a force of 1200 N is required for equilibrium to exist. The force acting on the disc will be 1200 + 400 = 1600 N. With a chair, as in Figure 4.6B, you are forced to sit in a position that causes the figure 15 cm to become smaller and thereby diminish the disc pressure.

This is because the back muscles must pull harder (static tension) when the body sits. Disc pressure is due to the bodyweight (mg) acting on the disc from above, and the contraction force (F) of the surrounding muscles (Figure 4.9).

The total compressing force in Figure 4.9 will be $mg + F$. Pressure (P) is calculated by dividing the force by the area of the disc. The L3 vertebra of an adult has an area of about 10 cm². The disc of a young person can withstand a stress of 800 kg, i.e. 8000 N. The ability of the discs of an older person to withstand stress is reduced to half of this. A young healthy disc can thus withstand a pressure of 800 N/cm². Compare these figures with those given on p. 92.

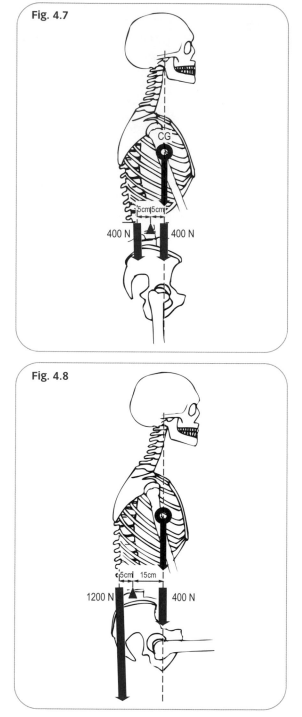

Fig. 4.7

5cm 5cm

400 N 400 N

CG

Fig. 4.8

5cm 15cm

1200 N 400 N

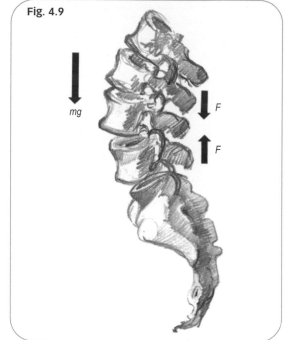

Fig. 4.9

mg

F

F

back muscles are stretched. For best results, 'hang' with bent hips (Figure 4.10) and support for your feet (relaxed iliopsoas = straight back).

As a matter of curiosity it can be mentioned that if the stress is of long duration, or very great, a certain amount of fluid can be pressed out of the nucleus pulposus and we can actually measure a shortening of body height. A weight-lifter may be several centimetres shorter after a heavy training session.

If we measure disc thickness after a night's rest, we will find that it is greater than if we measure it after a short period of normal activity.

When a person carries something heavy the disc pressure is, of course, increased. Asymmetrical stress produces greater pressure than symmetrical stress (p. 93). 'Hanging' from a bar reduces the pressure on the discs and thereby unloads the back. At the same time the

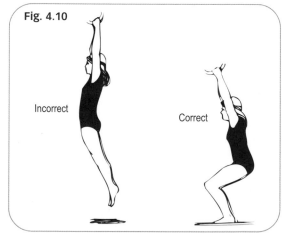

Fig. 4.10

Incorrect

Correct

Therefore, we are somewhat taller in the morning than at the middle of the day.

We become shorter as we get older because the vertebral discs shrink as the tissues degenerate.

There are many reasons for back pain. A common reason is that the annulus fibrosus tears and the nucleus pulposus is pressed backward, stretching the posterior longitudinal ligament, which runs posteriorly along the vertebral bodies in towards the spinal canal. If the ligament stretches, pain is felt via its pain-sensitive cells. (There are only a very few nerves to register pain in the torn disc.) This type of pain can cease if the back ceases to be stressed by the lifting of heavy objects, leaning forwards while working, or sitting still. If the nucleus pulposus bulges too far out, it can press against the nerve root, which passes through the intervertebral foramen. Pain is then felt from the muscles that are supplied by this nerve. Thus, pain can be felt in the shoulder when a cervical disc is injured. Tense muscles, small vertebral displacements, or worn-down intervertebral cartilage can put the same pressure on the nerves, thereby causing pain. If the pain is felt in the leg, the name sciatica is used to describe it because the irritated nerve in this case is called the sciatic nerve.

Some of the nerves that pass out from the intervertebral foramen and into a muscle can be drawn out a little further by stretching the muscle. This can cause the nerve to be pressed against a protrusion on the disc, producing severe pain in the leg. One way to examine a person to see if his sciatic nerve is irritated, is to place him on his back and lift his leg as shown in Figure 4.11. This test is called the Lasègués test. This type of pain must not be confused with that felt by stiff people who try to stretch their hamstrings (p. 69).

The annulus consists mainly of collagenous fibres, which stretch if they are subjected to prolonged stress. Hernia (tearing) is commonly caused by working in a position that subjects the disc to such stress for a long period of time. Lifting heavy objects increases disc pressure, which causes pressure in the nucleus pulposus to rupture the annulus fibrosus (Figure 4.12; top view).

The increased pressure produced by simultaneously lifting something heavy and twisting the trunk (e.g. shovelling earth) is greatest in the

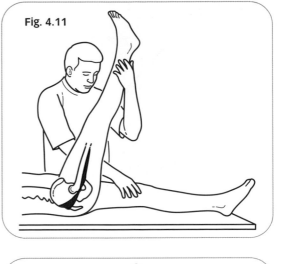

Fig. 4.11

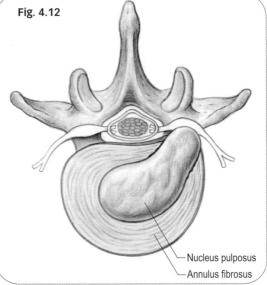

Fig. 4.12

Nucleus pulposus
Annulus fibrosus

posterior part of the disc, which is not protected by extra ligaments. Such activities are therefore especially dangerous for those who suffer from back complaints.

Using the moment of force law (p. 39), we can calculate which stresses the spinal column is subjected to in different positions, weight lifts and training exercises. The person in the example below (Figure 4.13) weighs 80 kg, of which 40 kg lies above the level of L3. Distance is measured in centimetres and force is measured in newtons. Thus, 40 kg corresponds to 400 N.

When lifting an object it is important to stand so that the external lever arm (the distance from L3 to the point where the force of gravity acts on

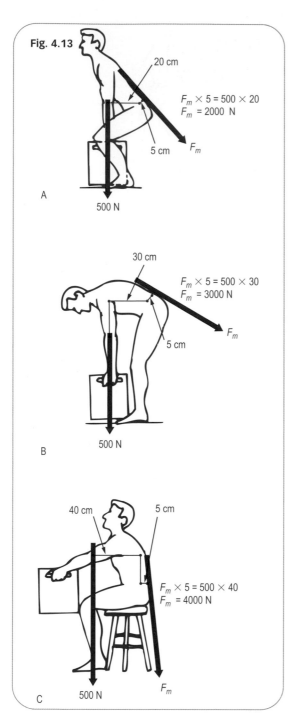

Fig. 4.13

A

20 cm

$F_m \times 5 = 500 \times 20$
$F_m = 2000$ N

5 cm

F_m

500 N

B

30 cm

$F_m \times 5 = 500 \times 30$
$F_m = 3000$ N

5 cm

F_m

500 N

C

40 cm

5 cm

$F_m \times 5 = 500 \times 40$
$F_m = 4000$ N

500 N

F_m

When he lifts from a sitting position (C), even very small weights subject his back to great loads.

According to the calculations above, the pressure to which the disc is subjected by the muscles in (C), is half of what it can tolerate in a healthy condition (8000 N, p. 89). This is true even when a person lifts a 'mere' 10 kg from a sitting position. The discs are, however, unloaded when a person instinctively tenses his abdominal muscles plus his diaphragm (p. 105). By doing so, he builds up the pressure in his abdomen, which has a piston effect in an upward and downward direction (preventing collapse). The disc – which is a part of the abdominal cavity's back wall – is thus protected. Hence, the pressure produced by the back muscles can be reduced by about 40% (Figure 4.14).

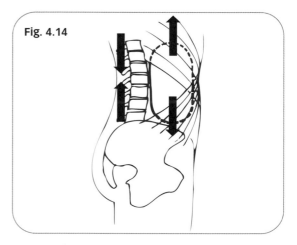

Fig. 4.14

The calculations above show how important it is to have well-trained abdominal muscles to unload the back, and strong leg muscles in order to lift correctly, i.e. with bent knees.

If a load can be distributed symmetrically by carrying it with both hands, the stress to which the back is subjected is considerably reduced compared with carrying with only one hand.

In Figures 4.15 and 4.16, the body weighs 40 kg above the level of L3. The load is 30 kg. The lever arm of the back muscles (for sideways bending) is 5 cm. In the symmetric lift, shown in Figure 4.15, the total work load is 700 N (150 N + 150 N + 400 N). When viewing this figure the reader should also take account of the discussion accompanying Figure 4.9. In the asymmetric lift, shown

both the body and the object) is as short as possible. In the example (Figure 4.13), the upper body (40 kg) + load (10 kg) is equal to 500 N. The back muscles are at work about 5 cm behind L3. When a person stands correctly (A), his external moment arm is about 20 cm, compared with 30 cm when he stands and lifts incorrectly (B).

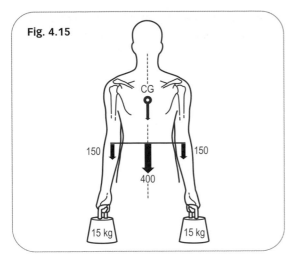

Fig. 4.15

150   150
400
15 kg   15 kg

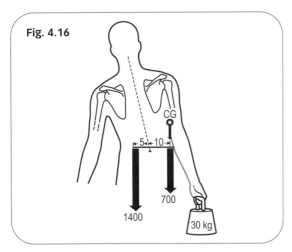

Fig. 4.16

CG
5 10
700
1400
30 kg

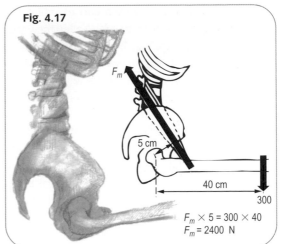

Fig. 4.17

F_m
5 cm
40 cm
300
$F_m \times 5 = 300 \times 40$
$F_m = 2400$ N

in Figure 4.16, suppose the centre of the body plus load falls 10 cm to the side of L3 (note that the common centre of gravity (CG) lies to the right of L3, even if the body tilts to the left). The back muscles must then contract with a force of:

$$F_m \times 5 = 700 \times 10$$

$$F_m = 1400 \text{ N}.$$

Total load is:

$$700 \text{ N} + 1400 \text{ N} = 2100 \text{ N}.$$

The back is heavily loaded when the iliopsoas (p. 58) is forced to work. The muscles are required to act statically to hold the legs straight out in front of a person who is hanging from a bar. If he weighs 80 kg, his legs weigh 30 kg, the centre of gravity of his legs lies 40 cm from his hip joint, and his iliopsoas operates with a lever arm of about 5 cm, then the force can be calculated as in Figure 4.17.

About 1100 N of this force acts to increase the curvature of the lumbar spine. The force pressing the discs together will be about 2200 N (Figure 4.18). If the abdominal muscles do not keep the back straight, then a force of 2200 N could greatly increase the pressure in certain parts of the disc.

Such an exercise is thus unsuitable for people with weak abdominal muscles. Some sporting events, however, subject the iliopsoas to considerably greater stress.

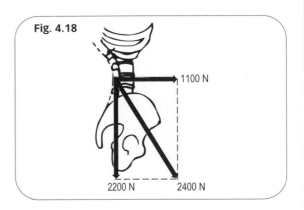

Fig. 4.18

1100 N
2200 N   2400 N

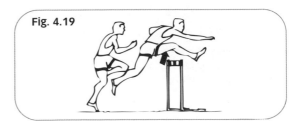

Fig. 4.19

By way of comparison we can examine the forces that are necessary to swing a leg forwards during running, jumping, hurdling, etc. (Figure 4.19). The weight and acceleration (for which the iliopsoas is responsible) of the leg may cause the force of muscle contraction to reach about 4000 N.

When we consider exercises that engage the back muscles, we must also take account of the stabilizing effect of the abdominal muscles. The diagrams that follow illustrate the different types of back and abdominal muscles found in the body.

Muscles of the back (erector spinae)

The muscles of the back can be classified schematically as follows.

1. Long back muscles (pass at least seven vertebrae).
2. Back muscles of average length (pass two to six vertebrae).
3. Short back muscles (go to the nearest vertebra).

The long muscles lie outermost (Figure 4.20). They are called:

- Iliocostalis (from the hip bone to the ribs).
- Longissimus (from the spinous processes to the transverse processes and ribs).
- Spinalis (between spinous processes).

The back muscles of average length (Figure 4.21) are:

- Semispinalis (passes four to seven vertebrae).
- Multifidus (passes two to three vertebrae).

The short muscles passing from vertebra to vertebra (Figure 4.22) are:

- Intertransversarii (between transverse processes).
- Interspinalis (between spinous processes).
- Rotatores (rotators) (between spinous and transverse processes).

The muscles work together as a unit. The iliocostalis, however, is more adapted for taking part in sideways bending than the remaining muscles. The most important muscles for turning the trunk are the rotators. A combination of bending and turning is important for all types of throwing (Figure 4.23).

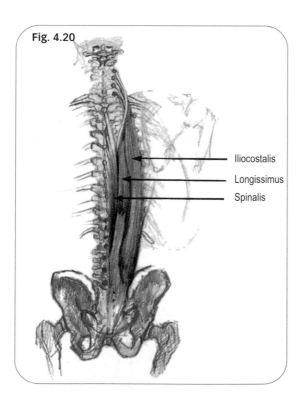

Fig. 4.20

Iliocostalis
Longissimus
Spinalis

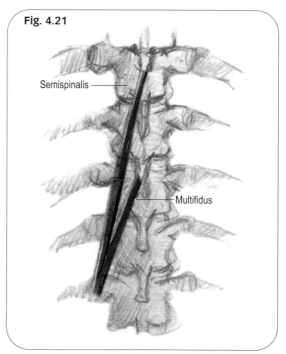

Fig. 4.21

Semispinalis

Multifidus

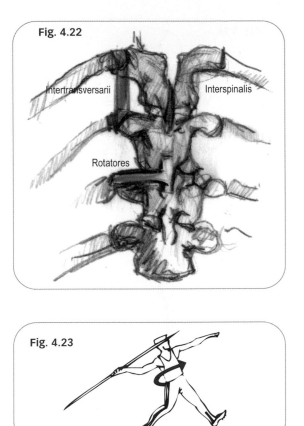

Fig. 4.22

Intertransversarii

Interspinalis

Rotatores

Fig. 4.23

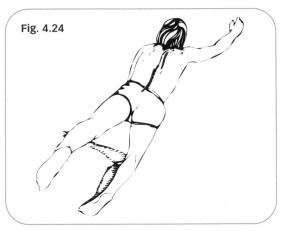

Fig. 4.24

activates the diagonal muscles that prevent the right shoulder and left hip from falling downwards. You should remain in that position for a few seconds so the muscles can work statically. Next, change positions by lifting your left arm and right leg (Figure 4.24).

It is believed that cramps of the short muscles – in particular the rotatores – are the most common cause of so-called lumbago. If cramp occurs in one muscle, the muscles surrounding it contract to prevent movements that could tear it. This, in turn, cuts off the blood supply to the area, causing cramp in other muscles.

Cramp can be relieved by taking the load off the muscles (bedrest) and inducing relaxation (warmth, massage, muscle-relaxing medication). Cramp may result from overexertion, unaccustomed movements or minor vertebral displacements caused by sudden stresses. The best protection is well-functioning back and abdominal musculature.

Exercises for the back

In the following exercise the rotatores are forced to work. Kneel on all fours; then, simultaneously lift your right arm and left leg (Figure 4.24). This

Additional exercises for the back are given below, along with the effect they are considered to have.

Figure 4.25A. This exercise should be done slowly. Well-trained young people can also turn sideways from the raised position in order to activate the rotators. The load to which the lower back is subjected can be increased by holding the arms stretched out in front of the body. Do not exaggerate backward bending of the neck. Do not go too far.

Figure 4.25B. Lift one leg at a time to train the hamstrings, the gluteus maximus (large buttock muscle) and the lower back musculature. Do the exercise slowly. *Stop* in the raised position for static training. In order to control speed do not combine exercises A and B.

Figure 4.25C. Lie on a vaulting horse with your pelvis free as shown in the diagram. Keeping your back straight, pull yourself up until you reach the horizontal plane. You will be training all your back muscles statically; your hip extensors concentrically on the way up, and eccentrically on the way down. You can vary the load with the help of your arms – little stress when your arms are by your sides, great stress when your arms are folded behind your neck. Light weights can be used.

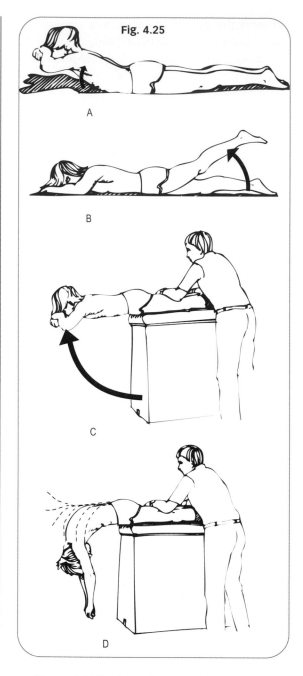

Fig. 4.25

A

B

C

D

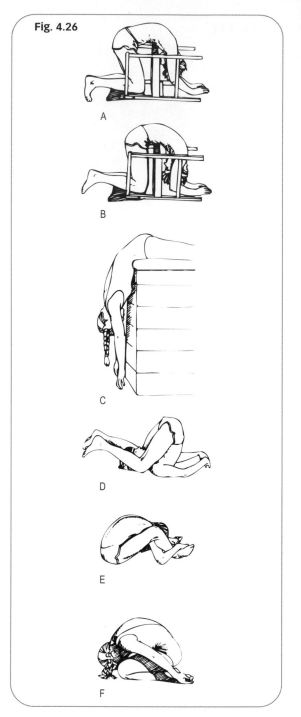

Fig. 4.26

A

B

C

D

E

F

Figure 4.25D. As in C except that you should roll up to the horizontal plane one vertebra at a time beginning at the lumbar spine. Your back muscles are then forced to work concentrically (in the order L5, L4, ..., C1) while rolling up, and eccentrically while rolling down (C1, ..., L5). The diagrams in Figure 4.26 show how the back muscles can be stretched by leaning forwards without subjecting the back to stress, so that the whole musculature can relax.

These positions also reduce disc pressure by pulling on the back (traction).

When training the back muscles (Figure 4.27) one can (1) allow the trunk to fall forward – keeping the legs and back straight – until the horizontal plane is reached. Then (2) in an easy

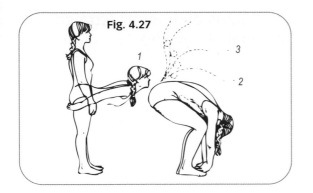

Fig. 4.27

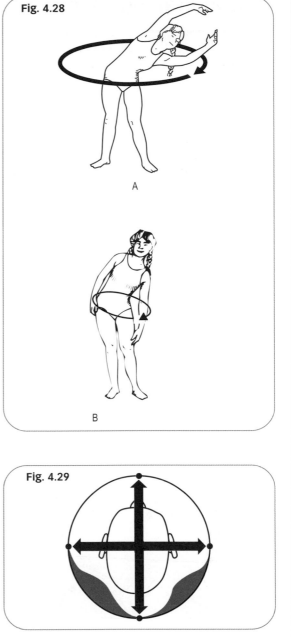

Fig. 4.28

A

B

Fig. 4.29

movement, bend further forwards with flexed knees and back.

Next, (3) roll up one vertebra at a time, beginning at the lumbar spine. The first phase (1) stresses the muscles of the back statically. The load increases as you approach the horizontal plane. You can increase the stress still further by making some 'breast strokes' with your arms while you are in the horizontal plane. By doing so, you will be shifting the centre of gravity of your upper body even farther away from your hips. By falling forwards beyond the horizontal plane, you can decrease the load for your back muscles (the load will instead be borne by the posterior longitudinal ligament, p. 89). People with back complaints and elderly people should avoid this.

Rolling up (see (3) in Figure 4.27) forces the back muscles to work concentrically along the entire length of the spine (compare Figure 4.25D). We are often told that rolling the trunk is a dangerous exercise, but there is no evidence that this is so. Moreover, trunk rolling exercises (Figure 4.28A) are often confused with hula-hula movements (Figure 4.28B).

Trunk rolling can be done by moving the upper body (trunk) in large circles while keeping the hips and legs still. If this movement is performed when the body is warmed up and if the pace is controlled, then there is no risk associated with it. By the same token, it can hardly be claimed to have especially beneficial effects.

Hula-hula movements increase the flexibility of the hip joints. Here, the feet and head are kept still while the hips are moved around in a circle.

As far as the neck is concerned, so-called head rolls should be avoided. There is a certain risk of doing these too quickly and thereby subjecting

the ligaments and cartilage to wear and tear. Figure 4.29 shows the approximate range of movement of the head. The head cannot bend as far obliquely backwards as it can in all other directions. The shaded regions of the diagram mark the dangerous areas through which the head may be forced to pass if it rolls around quickly. However, if you roll slowly and under control, you may follow the outer limits of the cervical spine's range of motion without any problems.

Abdominal muscles

As we have seen when examining movements that strain the back, a well-functioning abdominal musculature unloads the back during lifting, and stabilizes the spinal column (i.e. the abdominal muscles are antagonists to the back muscles). The example given on p. 92 show that the back muscles are always trained during lifting, standing, sitting, etc. The majority of people have abdominal muscles that are too weak in relation to their back muscles. Thus, general abdominal muscle training (Figure 4.30A) can be recommended for everyone. Athletes should strengthen their abdominal muscles with exercises that subject them to a heavy load (Figure 4.30B). After that they should train their hip flexors (iliopsoas, rectus femoris (straight thigh muscle)) and back extensors for strength. (For such exercises, see pp. 58 and 95.)

In order to judge correctly which exercises to choose and how to execute them, we must first understand how the abdominal muscles function. It is also important to familiarize ourselves with the connection that exists between the back, abdomen and hip flexors.

There are four different kinds of abdominal muscle:

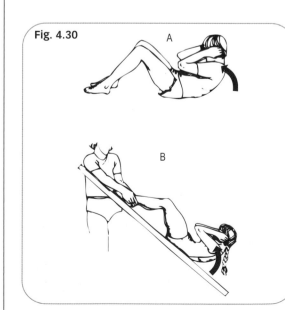

Fig. 4.30

(A) Rectus abdominis (straight abdominal muscle) (Figure 4.31)

The rectus abdominis originates from the apex of the sternum (breastbone) and is inserted into the upper part of the pubic part of the hip bone. When it contracts, the body bends forwards at the lumbar and thoracic spines. If you lie on your back (as in Figure 4.30A) and pull your upper body up as far as possible without tipping your pelvis forward (no movement at the hip joint), then you will maximally shorten your straight abdominal muscle.

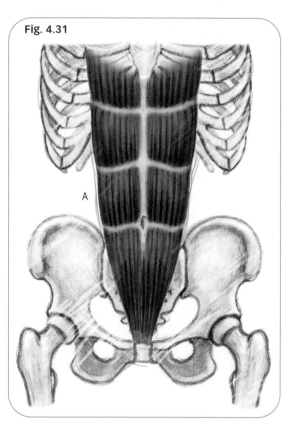

Fig. 4.31

(B) Obliquus externus abdominis (external oblique abdominal muscle) (Figure 4.32)

The obliquus externus abdominis arises from the anterior inferior part of the chest (lower ribs). This muscle becomes an aponeurosis (a tendinous sheet) that covers the rectus abdominis above, and below it is inserted into the iliac crest (crest of the hip bone) and inguinal (groin) ligament. In the lower part of the abdomen the aponeuroses of the left and right obliquus externus abdominis meet.

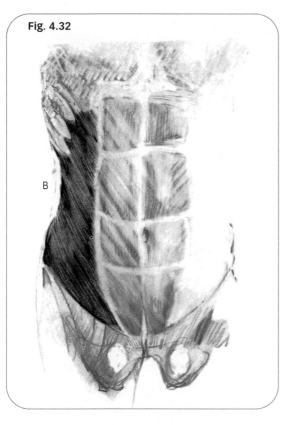

Fig. 4.32

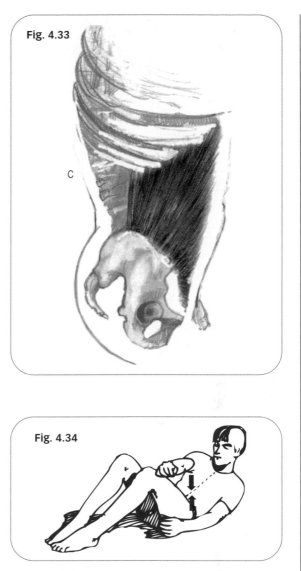

Fig. 4.33

Fig. 4.34

(C) Obliquus internus abdominis (internal oblique abdominal muscle) (Figure 4.34)

The obliquus internus abdominis arises from the hip bone and inguinal (groin) ligament, becomes an aponeurosis (a tendinous sheet) passing under the rectus abdominis (straight abdominal muscle), and is inserted into the linea alba (the fibrous band that runs down between the two rectus abdominis muscles (straight abdominal muscles)).

The oblique abdominal muscles act to assist the rectus abdominis. In addition, they can turn the trunk. In diagonal sit-ups (Figure 4.33), the stress to which the oblique abdominal muscles are subjected will increase with the result that if the right shoulder is turned towards the left hip, the right external and left internal oblique muscles will be engaged.

(D) Transversus abdominis (transverse abdominal muscle) (Figure 4.35)

The transversus abdominis is not connected with any movements. It only affects the figure (see

Figure 4.36) by pulling the abdomen in. It is also brought into action when the abdominal pressure is increased by so-called abdominal presses. All the abdominal muscles can, upon contraction, increase abdominal pressure (which would try to widen the abdominal cavity). In this way, the discs are unloaded during lifting (p. 92).

Figure 4.37 shows a horizontal cross-section of the body. From it we can detect the relationship between the back and abdominal muscles.

(E) Quadratus lumborum (square lumbar muscle) (Figure 4.38)

Here, we should also mention the most important sideways flexor. Its name is quadratus lumborum (p. 101). It takes part in sideways bending

Fig. 4.35

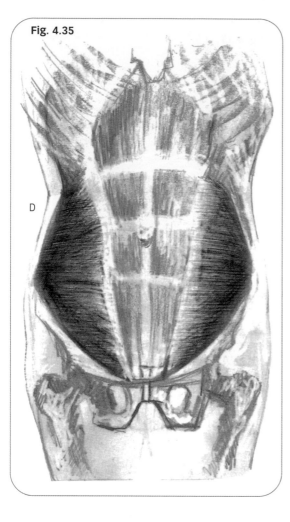

D

Fig. 4.36

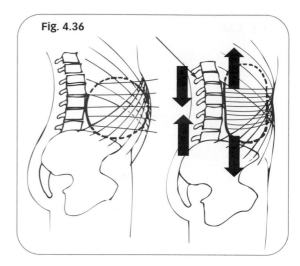

when the movement occurs at the lumbar spine (Figure 4.39). Compare this with the movements described on p. 57 that take place at the hip and also engage the abductor muscles.

When a person lies on their back, there is a certain curvature on the lumbar spine that is due to the natural curvature of the spine as well as tension in the iliopsoas. The back can be pressed to the floor (Figure 4.40B) by using the abdominal muscles (**a**), buttock muscles (**b**), and hamstrings (**h**) to tip the pelvis backwards. This would be found easier to do if the knees were bent and the head lifted a little (Figure 4.41).

Fig. 4.37

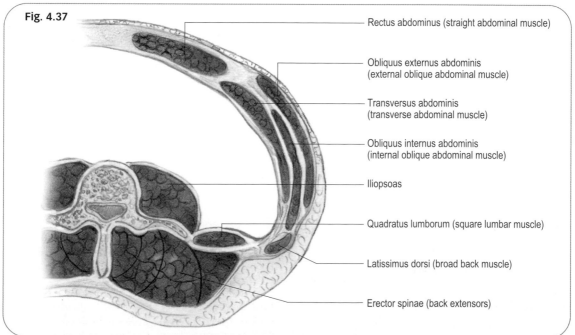

Rectus abdominus (straight abdominal muscle)

Obliquus externus abdominis (external oblique abdominal muscle)

Transversus abdominis (transverse abdominal muscle)

Obliquus internus abdominis (internal oblique abdominal muscle)

Iliopsoas

Quadratus lumborum (square lumbar muscle)

Latissimus dorsi (broad back muscle)

Erector spinae (back extensors)

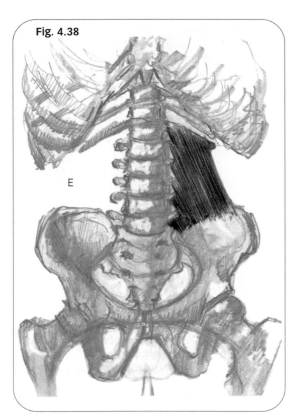

Fig. 4.38

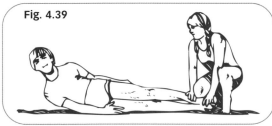

Fig. 4.39

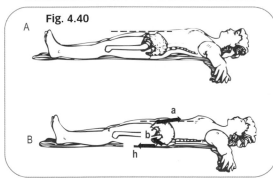

Fig. 4.40

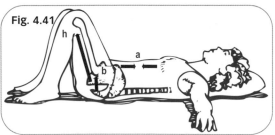

Fig. 4.41

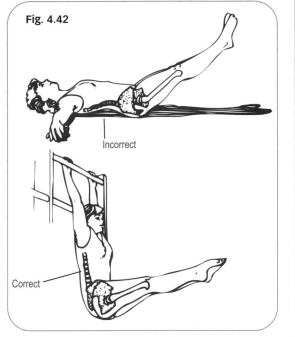

Fig. 4.42

Thus, the iliopsoas has been relaxed and a forward bending of the spine initiated.

If you lie on your back and lift your legs, keeping them straight, you will easily reach a position where your back curvature is considerably greater than it is in a standing position (Figure 4.42). This is because the force with which the iliopsoas lifts the legs also acts on the back in such a way that the curvature is increased (see p. 93 (Figure 4.18)).

Exercises that require a person to lift straight legs, or give resistance to hip flexion (p. 60), should only be undertaken if the abdominal muscles are capable of stabilizing the back (tipping the pelvis). Such exercises should be left to those who are relatively well trained. Their aim, strictly speaking, is to strengthen the hip flexors. Nevertheless, there is a static training effect from which the abdominal muscles benefit.

If a person wants to train only their abdominal muscles, they should make sure that movement takes place at the spine and not at the hips. The most common exercise for strengthening the abdominal muscles is the sit-up. The best way to prevent a sit-up from recruiting the iliopsoas is to be so bent at the hip that the muscle cannot contract with any degree of force. A common mistake is to bend the knees (with

101

accompanying hip bending) at the same time as the feet are held under a wall-bar. In this position, the hip is not bent enough to disengage the iliopsoas and, because the feet are supported, the body can sit up without any great effort on the part of the abdominal muscles. If you assume the position shown in Figure 4.43 – without supporting your feet – you must roll up vertebra by vertebra (i.e. engage your abdominal muscles) before you bend your hip and thereby pull yourself up.

The best way to train your abdominal muscles is by strongly flexing your hip, making sure that your feet are unsupported. It is then only possible to do half a sit-up (i.e. maximal contraction of your abdominal muscles) without bending your hips further.

If you remain in the raised position and rotate to each side, you will be training your rectus abdominis (straight abdominal muscle) statically as well as increasing the load on your oblique abdominal muscles. You can vary the quantity of exercise by keeping your arms straight by your sides (easy), crossing your arms over your chest or placing your hands over your ears (difficult) (Figure 4.44). The work load can be further increased by adding weights.

When we consider how the external stress increases during a sit-up (Figure 4.45), we see

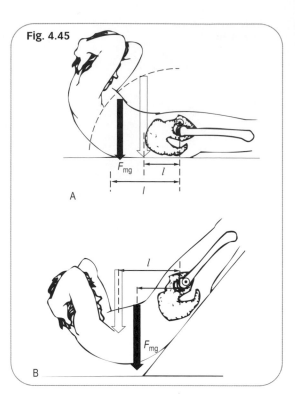

Fig. 4.45

A

B

that the centre of gravity of the upper body lies some way from the hip joint at the beginning of the exercise, and that this distance decreases as the body rolls up vertebra by vertebra (Figure 4.45A). External stress ($F_{mg} \times l$) decreases as the abdominal muscles contract.

If a person lies on a sloping plane, the external stress will increase as he pulls himself up and as his abdominal muscles shorten (i.e. weaken). He would thus find this exercise very demanding (Figure 4.45B).

Which of the following is the most demanding: sitting up on a slanting bench (45° slope) or sitting up from the floor with 10 kg on your chest? Try them!

A person exercising on a slanting plane must have support for his feet. This means that he is tempted to use his iliopsoas at an early stage instead of rolling one vertebra at a time (i.e. working his abdominal muscles).

The four following examples are designed to illustrate the relationship between external forces (the weight of the legs and upper body) and internal forces (contractions of iliopsoas and abdominal muscles).

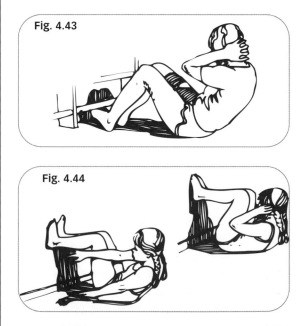

Fig. 4.43

Fig. 4.44

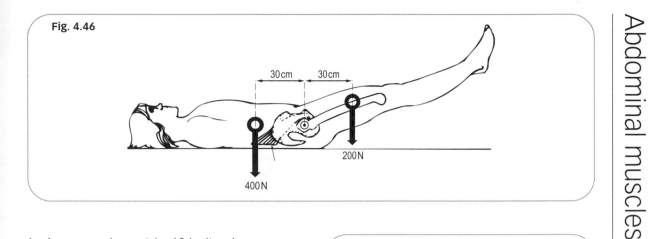

Fig. 4.46

30 cm 30 cm

400 N

200 N

1. A person who weighs 60 kg lies down as shown in Figure 4.46. The centre of gravity of his upper body, which weighs about 40 kg, is presumed to lie 30 cm above his hip joint. His legs weigh 20 kg. Their centre of gravity lies 30 cm below the hip. Thus, according to the formula, $M = F \times l$, where M represents the moment of force of the upper body,

$M = 400 \times 30 = 12\ 000$ Ncm.

The moment of force of the legs,

$M = 200 \times 30 = 6\ 000$ Ncm.

2. The iliopsoas (the main muscle group responsible for hip flexion) is presumed to be positioned so that its direction of pull in relation to the hip is 6 cm (Figure 4.47). If its contraction force reaches 1000 N, then the moment of force acting on the leg will be $1000 \times 6 = 6000$ Ncm (i.e. equal to the moment of force of the legs, according to Figure 4.46). He can thus begin to lift his legs. If the muscle force is even greater, he can lift his legs with greater speed.

3. If his legs are fixed and the iliopsoas contracts with a force of 2000 N, then the muscle's moment of force will be $2000 \times 6 = 12000$ Ncm and he can lift his upper body (as shown in Figure 4.48).

4. In order to sit up without supporting his legs, he must roll up one vertebra at a time using his abdominal muscles until the centre of gravity of his upper body lies 15 cm (instead of 30 cm) from his hip

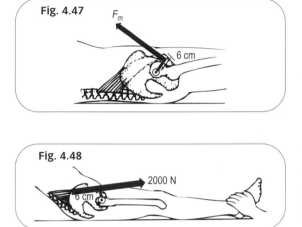

Fig. 4.47 F_m

6 cm

Fig. 4.48

2000 N

6 cm

(Figure 4.49). The iliopsoas will now lift both his upper body and his legs. By bending a little further forwards at the spine, he can sit up without moving his legs. If his legs are bent, and they are unsupported, his abdominal muscles will be forced to work over an even greater distance before his hips can be bent.

The diagrams in Figure 4.50 present some variations of abdominal muscle training. You should make sure that movement takes place at your spine (easy forward bending) before possible movements take place at your hip joint. Never subject your legs to more stress than your abdominal musculature (whose job it is to hold your back slightly bent forward) can cope with.

There is rarely ever a need of stretching exercises for the abdominal muscles. Usually the vertebrae restrict movements backwards, not shortened abdominals.

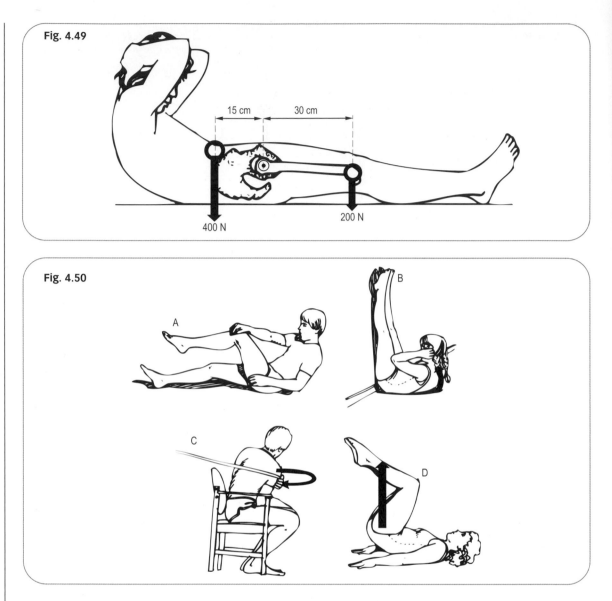

Fig. 4.49

15 cm   30 cm

400 N   200 N

Fig. 4.50

A   B

C   D

Respiratory muscles

Here we will consider the structure of the rib cage and function of the breathing musculature in outline only. The reader is referred to the literature on physiology for a deeper study.

The rib cage (Figure 4.51) consists of 12 ribs (or costae). The first 10 (from the top) are attached directly (first seven) or indirectly to the sternum (breast bone) via costal cartilages. Rib numbers 11 and 12 have no anterior attachment and are therefore called floating ribs.

The chest and abdominal cavities are separated by the most important muscle of respiration, the diaphragm. This muscle arises from the lumbar vertebrae, from the lower ribs, and from the xiphoid process, which is at the bottom of the sternum. The diaphragm arches up like a dome into the chest cavity (Figure 4.52). When the muscle fibres contract, they become less arched and thus cause the central tendinous part of the dome to descend. During contraction, the volume of the chest cavity increases (inspiration) and the volume of the abdominal cavity decreases. The abdomen thus bulges out, which is why this type of breathing is called abdominal breathing (deep breathing).

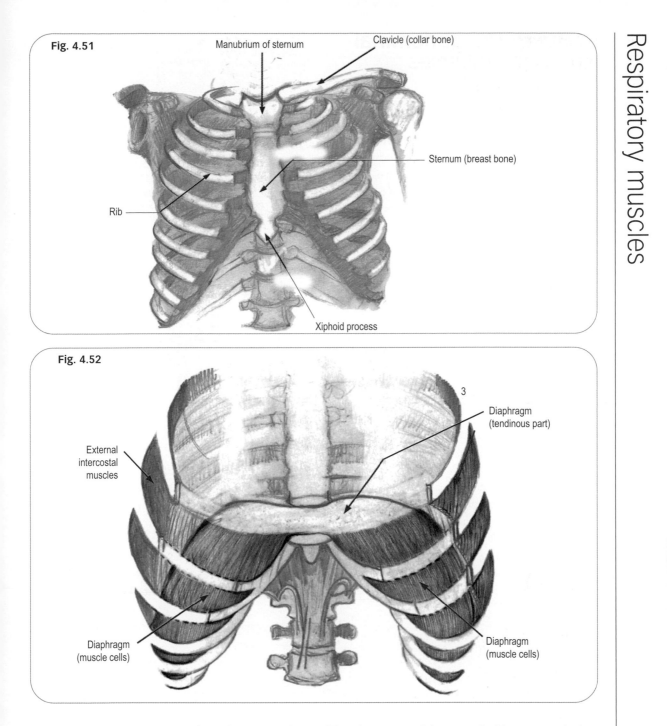

Fig. 4.51

Manubrium of sternum

Clavicle (collar bone)

Sternum (breast bone)

Rib

Xiphoid process

Fig. 4.52

3

Diaphragm (tendinous part)

External intercostal muscles

Diaphragm (muscle cells)

Diaphragm (muscle cells)

Besides functioning as a breathing muscle, the diaphragm assists the abdominal muscles in increasing intra-abdominal pressure. This is important when it comes to lifting heavy objects (see p. 100 (Figure 4.36)). The volume of the chest cavity can also be increased by raising the ribs. This is accomplished by the action of muscles that are attached to the ribs.

The direction of the muscle fibres is such that they lift the lower ribs up towards the upper ribs (3, in Figure 4.52). These muscles are called external intercostal muscles. This latter type of breathing is called chest breathing. A number of muscles (back, chest, neck, etc.) may exert an influence on the rib cage during forced breathing.

Training the abdominal and back muscles

When training the abdominal and back muscles you have to consider the fact that the construction of the vertebrae makes the spine act as a joint with three axes. You should have exercises for flexion–extension, side to side and rotations in both directions. Back muscles are postural (help keep us standing upright) and are therefore well trained compared with the abdominal muscles (Figure 4.53). The more inactive a human is the greater the difference in strength between the two groups. The abdominals are strained naturally when you lift, carry, run, chop wood, dig, shovel snow ... rare activities in today's society. We sometimes try to compensate for this lack of functional training by doing crunches and sit ups. Exercises completely strange to the human race. (How would it look like if we all of a sudden had to lie down on our backs to exercise to keep in shape in order to escape all sorts of predators?)

Pure flexion in the spine causes the tip of the sternum (breast bone) to move 10–15 cm towards the pubis (pubic bone). By contrast, movement in the hip joint has nothing to do with the abdominal muscles. When you choose your type of exercise you should decide whether you want to stress only the abdomen, only the hip flexors, or both. If your target is the abdomen you should have as much flexion in the hip joint as possible in order to prevent the

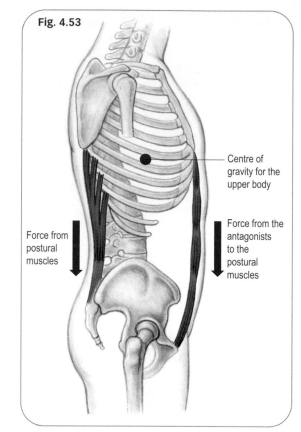

Fig. 4.53

Centre of gravity for the upper body

Force from postural muscles

Force from the antagonists to the postural muscles

hip muscles from assisting. Of the four positions in Figure 4.54, the strongest hip flexor (iliopsoas) has fewer and fewer possibilities to work as you change position from 1–4. A special trick is to press the heels against the surface (try to flex your knees). You do that with your hamstrings, a muscle group that at the same time tries to extend the hip joint. The effect of your

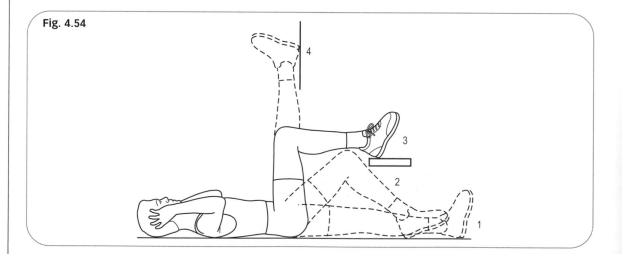

Fig. 4.54

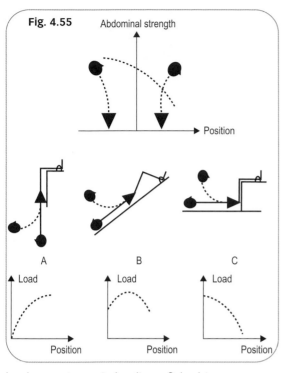

Fig. 4.55

Abdominal strength

Position

A   B   C

Load   Load   Load

Position   Position   Position

heel press is static loading of the hip extensors, which makes it almost impossible to activate the hip flexors at the same time. Try it!

The purpose of inactive flexors is to diminish painful forces in the lower back and to put all the stress on the abdomen. You want to do effective short crunches not complete sit-ups. With support above the feet you automatically activate the

hip flexors and you can sit up. You then train both muscle groups. You have to be strong enough in the abdomen to do this (see p. 60), otherwise you can get low back pain. The iliopsoas has a strong tendency to arch the lower back, something that should be prevented by the abdominal muscles. All exercises for the abdomen could and should be varied with different kinds of rotations.

The strength profile of the abdominal muscle group declines when you bend forward (Figure 4.55). Your strongest position is when you are slightly bent backwards and you are weak when bent forwards. To do sit ups in the three positions (A)–(C) in Figure 4.55 will have three different effects. The diagram shows how your abdomen is stressed. Position (C) is the one which coincides best with the strength profile. Position (A) is specialized for athletes having the desire to be strong in a crunched position (hurdlers, gymnasts, divers ...). With a disc weight held against your chest you can moderate the load.

A contracting muscle pulls with exactly the same force at both ends. Whether it moves at just one end or both depends on the circumstances. In an ordinary sit-up, it is the upper body that moves. If you block that part, the movement takes place in the lower body. In most cases you then need more force because the moment of force for the lower part is greater (Figure 4.56).

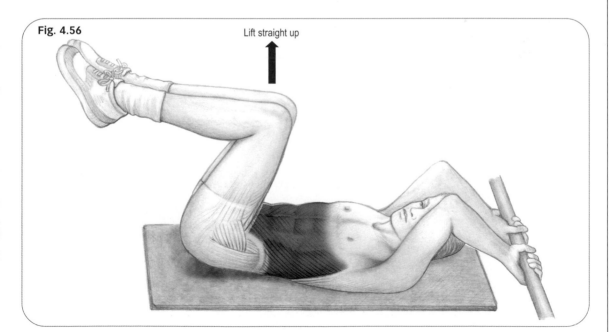

Fig. 4.56

Lift straight up

When training the back extensors you can have exactly the same type of discussion as for the abdomen. Simple extension activates the back (erector spinae) muscles, but the movement mostly combines with a hip extension as well (gluteus and hamstrings). The exercise in Figure 4.57 has been made more and more difficult (a)–(c) by changing the position of the arms, and adding a disc weight in (d).

Exercises moving from side to side and rotations are illustrated in Figures 4.58 and 4.59.

Moving from side to side with a barbell in the right hand puts strain on the left abdominals (Figure 4.58A).

In Figure 4.58B the upper body acts as load for the right abdominals. You can change the load by holding your arms in different positions. An extra weight behind the neck in position 2 gives a considerably higher load.

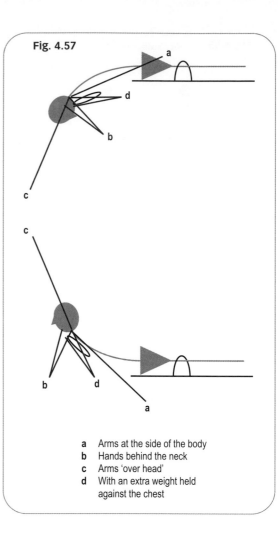

Fig. 4.57

a   Arms at the side of the body
b   Hands behind the neck
c   Arms 'over head'
d   With an extra weight held against the chest

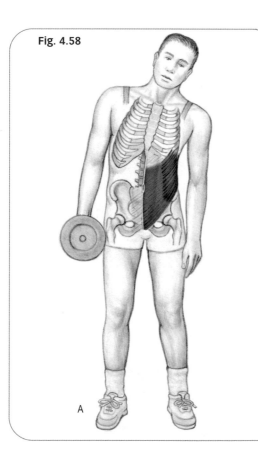

Fig. 4.58

A

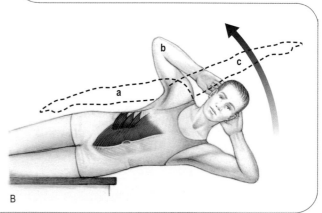

B

In Figure 4.59A your legs act as a load. Straight legs cause the centre of gravity of the legs to be further away from the spine and force the oblique abdominal muscles to work harder.

Rotation back and through, as in Figure 4.59B, with a barbell on the shoulder, is another way to exercise your obliques (and the rotational part of the back muscles). The inertia of the barbell acts as a load when it is accelerated and braked (see Chapter 6). Be very careful with this exercise. Use low weight and low speed until you are absolutely sure what you can carry out. If you cannot brake in time, there is a great risk of injury!

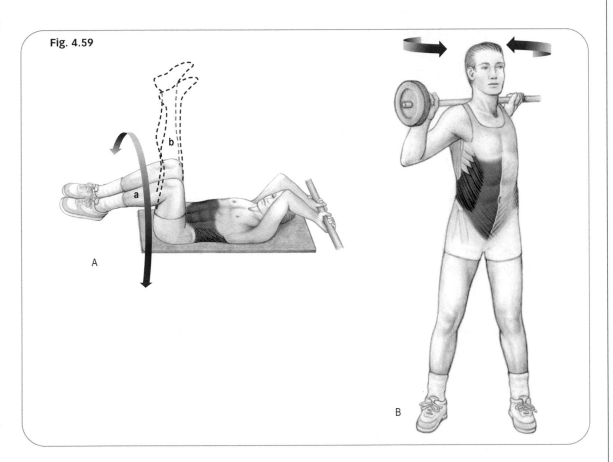

Fig. 4.59

Chapter 5

Anatomy and function of the arm

The movements of the upper arm are controlled by many muscles. Three different muscle groups are responsible for the movement of the shoulder joint. Figure 5.1 shows muscles from these three groups.

Group A. Muscles that have their origin on the scapula (shoulder blade) and that are inserted into the humerus (upper arm bone).

Group B. Muscles that have their origin on the trunk and their insertion on the scapula.

Group C. Muscles that have their origin on the trunk and their insertion on the humerus.

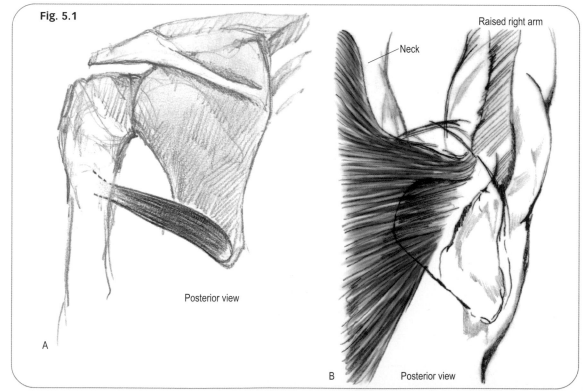

Fig. 5.1

Posterior view

A

Raised right arm

Neck

B   Posterior view

Fig. 5.1 cont'd

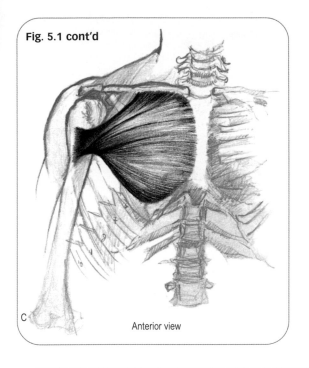

Anterior view

The scapula is triangular in form. This is illustrated in Figure 5.2, in which the left side is viewed from the back. A sharp spine (spine of the scapula) (1) projects backwards and forms two depressions on the posterior surface of the scapula. The outer end of the spine forms a flat roof (acromion) (2) overhanging the shoulder joint. The anterior part of the acromion articulates with the clavicle (collar bone) (3) at the acromioclavicular joint (outer collar bone joint) (4).

The sternoclavicular joint (inner collar bone joint) (5) (Figure 5.3, right-sided view from the front) articulates with the manubrium of the sternum (breastbone) (6). The outermost part of the scapula presents a shallow articular surface (glenoid cavity) (7) against which the humerus articulates (8). Not far from this joint, a little below the clavicle, is a bony projection that gives attachment to muscles,

Fig. 5.2

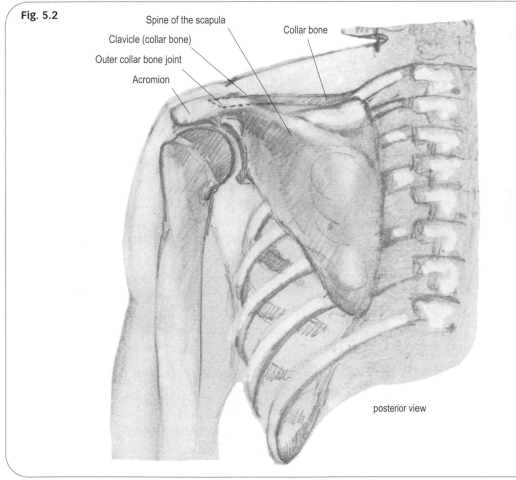

Spine of the scapula

Clavicle (collar bone)

Outer collar bone joint

Acromion

Collar bone

posterior view

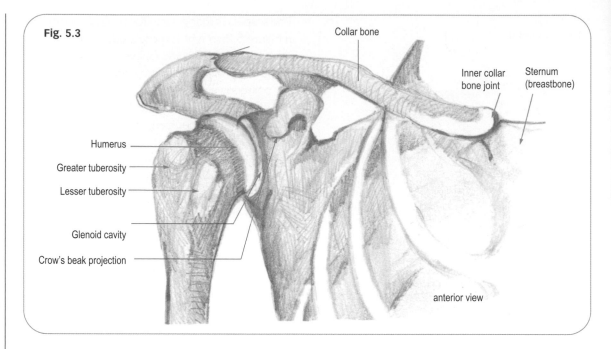

Fig. 5.3

Collar bone

Inner collar bone joint

Sternum (breastbone)

Humerus

Greater tuberosity

Lesser tuberosity

Glenoid cavity

Crow's beak projection

anterior view

including the most important elbow flexor, the biceps brachii (two-headed arm muscle). This process is called the coracoid process (crow's beak projection) (9).

The arm articulates with the scapula at a ball and socket joint, allowing the following movements, in all planes:

1. Forward and backward swings (flexion–extension).
2. Outward and inward swings (abduction–adduction).
3. Outward and inward turns (lateral and medial rotation).

Practically the whole of the scapula functions as an area of origin for muscles. Between the neck and the shaft of the humerus, we can distinguish two roughened projections of bone from which slight ridges run continuous with the shaft; the outer projection (greater tuberosity) (10) and the anterior projection (lesser tuberosity) (11), which, together with their ridges, will be referred to here simply as the external and anterior areas of attachment.

Many of the muscles of the scapula have Latin names only. Translations are given in parentheses.

Group A

Group A consists of the following five muscles:

1. Supraspinatus ('above-the-shoulder-blade-spine' muscle)

(Supra = above; spina = spine). This lifts (abducts) the arm and rotates it outwards. It lies below the large muscle that gives the shoulder its contour: the deltoideus (deltoid muscle) (p. 116). Figure 5.4 shows a left-sided view of the supraspinatus, which lies below the deltoideus, from the back.

2. Teres major (greater round muscle)

(Teres = smooth and rounded; major = greater). This large, rounded muscle brings the arm to the side (adducts) and rotates it inwards. It works with the latissimus dorsi muscle (broad back muscle) (p. 117) (Figure 5.5; viewed from behind).

3. Infraspinatus ('below-the-shoulder-blade-spine' muscle)

4. Teres minor (lesser round muscle)

In the gap between the supraspinatus and teres major, there are two muscles that together adduct the arm and rotate it outwards. These muscles

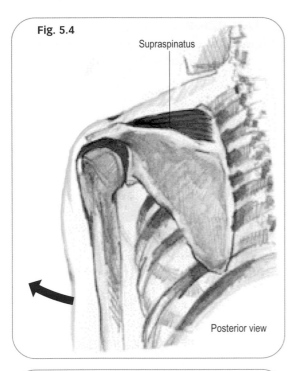

Fig. 5.4

Supraspinatus

Posterior view

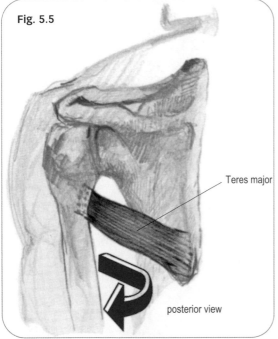

Fig. 5.5

Teres major

posterior view

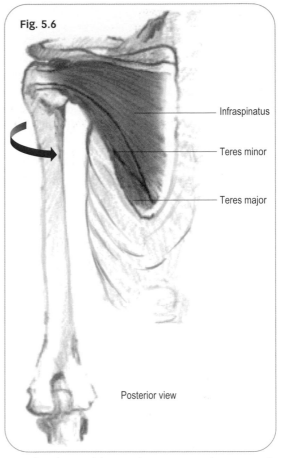

Fig. 5.6

Infraspinatus

Teres minor

Teres major

Posterior view

muscle that adducts the arm and rotates it inwards. Its name is subscapularis (sub = under; scapula = shoulder blade). If the position of the arm is blocked the muscle can adjust the position of the shoulder blade. Figure 5.7 shows the left shoulder viewed from the front.

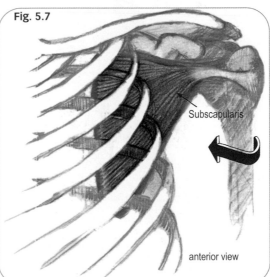

Fig. 5.7

Subscapularis

anterior view

are called infraspinatus (infra = below) and teres minor (minor = lesser, smaller). Figure 5.6 shows the left shoulder viewed from the back.

5. Subscapularis (anterior shoulder blade muscle)

Covering the inside of the scapula (shoulder blade) (against the back wall of the rib cage) is a

Group B

In order to move the arm with sufficient force, the articular surfaces of the scapula (shoulder blade) must be positioned in such a way that the arm has an optimal starting point for its movement. The scapula can be: elevated–depressed (10–12 cm), abducted–adducted (15 cm) and rotated outwards and inwards.

Outward rotation means that the articular surfaces of the scapula are directed outwards and upwards (see Figure 5.10).

The muscles that raise the scapula are:

1. Levator scapulae

(Levator = 'raiser').

2. Rhomboideus major and minor (greater and lesser rhomboid muscles)

Lifting and a certain inward rotation occur simultaneously (Figure 5.8; left side viewed from front). Both of the muscles below are covered by trapezius.

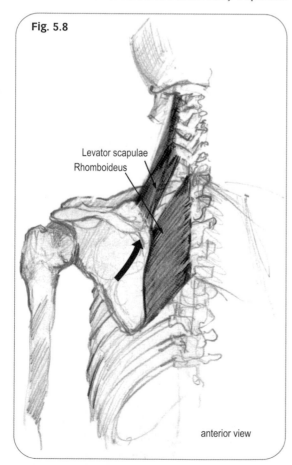

Fig. 5.8

Levator scapulae
Rhomboideus

anterior view

3. Trapezius (Figure 5.9)

Origin: base of the skull and the spines of the cervical and thoracic vertebrae.

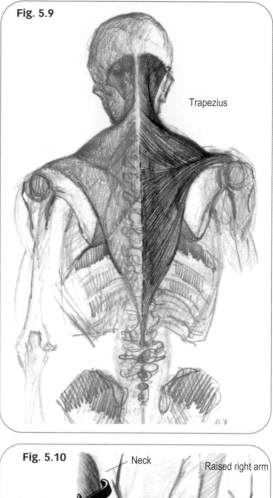

Fig. 5.9

Trapezius

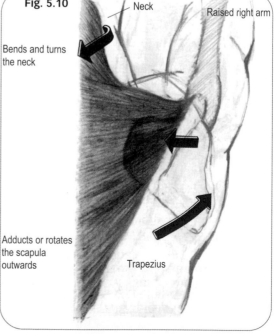

Fig. 5.10

Neck

Raised right arm

Bends and turns the neck

Adducts or rotates the scapula outwards

Trapezius

Insertion: spine of scapula (shoulder blade spine) and external part of the clavicle (collar bone).

Function: raises and adducts the scapula and rotates it outwards. Turns the head and bends the neck backwards (see Figure 5.10; right shoulder viewed from the back).

Group C

The large, flat, muscles that arise from the trunk and pass to the upper arm. They are the most important muscles for strength and flexibility.

1. Pectoralis major (greater chest muscle)

(Pectoris = chest)

Origin (Figure 5.11): (1) inner part of the clavicle (collar bone), (2) manubrium and body of the sternum (breastbone) and (3) part of the costal cartilage (of the ribs). (Also the aponeurosis of the obliquus externus abdominis (external oblique abdominal muscle).)

Insertion: external attachment area of the humerus (upper arm bone).

Function: forms the anterior wall of the armpit, and adducts the arm and rotates it inwards. It pulls a raised arm down and swings a lowered arm forwards (flexion of the shoulder). Exercises for the pectoralis major are shown below.

Lie on your back on a bench with dumbbells in your hands (Figure 5.12). Lift the dumbbells and keep your arms slightly bent in order to avoid overstraining your elbows. The upward movement provides concentric training, and the downward movement provides eccentric training. You can vary the load by varying the extent to which you bend your elbows. By keeping your arms a little straighter on the way down, you subject the muscle to a little more stress.

Figure 5.13 shows a variation of the exercise in Figure 5.12. This exercise trains only the upper part of the muscle (1 in Figure 5.11) namely, that part which has its origin on the clavicle (i.e. prevents the arm from falling downwards). Other muscles taking part in the exercise are the deltoideus (deltoid muscle) (see Figure 5.17A–B) and biceps brachii (two-headed arm muscle) (see Figure 5.26A–C).

Bending and stretching the arms (push-ups) while the hands are well separated activates

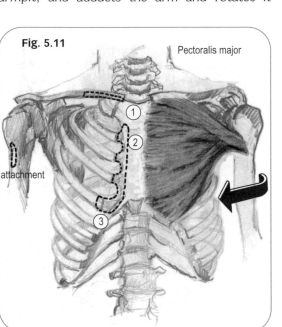

Fig. 5.11

Pectoralis major

attachment

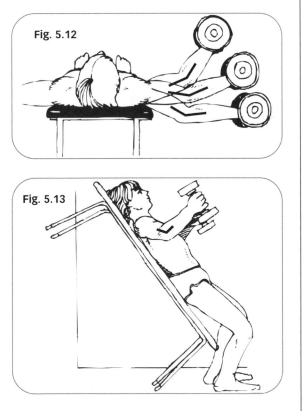

Fig. 5.12

Fig. 5.13

pectoralis major, and also triceps brachii (three-headed arm muscle), deltoideus, serratus anterior (anterior serrated muscle) and trapezius.

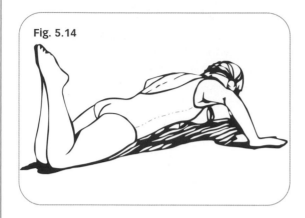

Fig. 5.14

Static training is provided if you press the palms of your hands hard together for a couple of seconds. Hold your hands low in front of you in order to activate the part of pectoralis that has its origin at 3 in Figure 5.11. Hands right in front of the chest moves the stress up to 2. Hands over your head activates 1.

A good way to round off these exercises is to stretch the pectoralis major following the PNF

Fig. 5.15

A

B

(proprioceptive neuromuscular facilitation) method (Figure 5.15A and B).

2. Deltoideus (deltoid muscle)

(Figure 5.16A and B)

Origin: outer part of the clavicle (collar bone), and along the entire spine of the posterior surface of the scapula (shoulder blade). (May even be assigned to group A.)

Insertion: deltoid tuberosity of the humerus (along the shaft of the upper arm bone).

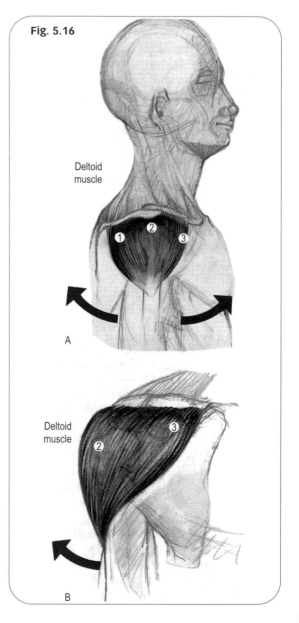

Fig. 5.16

Deltoid
muscle

A

Deltoid
muscle

B

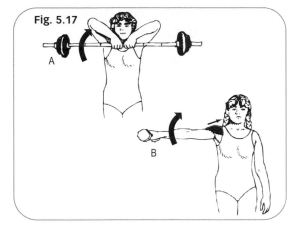

Fig. 5.17

Function: since its origin arches around the shoulder joint, this muscle can take part in all the movements of the arms. Its most important function is to (2) lift the arm straight outwards and upwards (abduction). The parts of the muscle that arise from the posterior surface of the scapula (1) swing the arms backwards and rotate it outwards. The parts that arise from the clavicle (3) swing the arm forwards and rotate it inwards.

The deltoideus is trained in almost all exercises that involve the arm. By lifting as shown in Figure 5.17, you can train the entire muscle. The weights in (B) should not exceed your ability to lift – with almost straight arms – the full distance six to eight times. Lift and lower your arms at the same pace; supraspinatus ('above-the-shoulder-blade-spine' muscle) is also trained in this exercise, see Figure 5.4.

3. Latissimus dorsi (broad back muscle)

(Latus =side, flank; dorsum = slope of hill) (Figure 5.18; right side viewed from the back).

Origin: the spine of the lower half of the spinal column down to the sacrum and, from it, out to the iliac crest (crest of the hip bone).

Insertion: anterior attachment area of the humerus (upper arm bone).

Function: forms the back wall of the armpit and pulls the arm in behind the back (i.e. swings it backwards and rotates the humerus inwards).

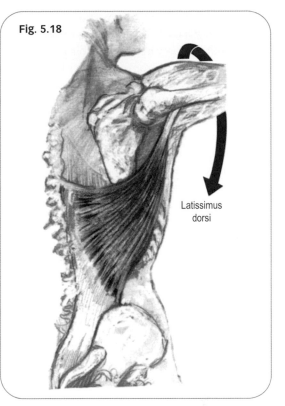

Fig. 5.18

Latissimus dorsi

There is equipment for training the latissimus dorsi in the majority of bodybuilding gymnasia. Using the special latissimus training apparatus (Figure 5.19A), you should be able to repeat the exercise about six to eight times by using the weights.

By pulling yourself up so that your head comes in front of the bar (Figure 5.19B), you will train exactly the same muscles as in (A), but with a greater effort (total bodyweight). The biceps brachii (two-headed arm muscle) (arm bending), trapezius (shoulder blade positioning) and the pectoralis major (greater chest muscle) (upper arm adduction) also take part in this exercise.

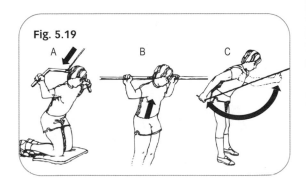

Fig. 5.19

117

Figure 5.19C shows how you can train the latissimus dorsi by pulling on a suspended weight with a rubber hose. In general, this muscle does not need flexibility training. If you bend forcefully to one side and hold your arms outstretched above your head, you may possibly feel the latissimus blocking the movement.

The exercises below (Figures 5.20 and 5.21) give examples of pure shoulder rotation.

Lie on your stomach on a bench with your elbows pointing outwards (Figure 5.20), and lift a dumbbell backwards (inward rotation of the shoulder) and forwards (outward rotation of the shoulder).

The main muscles helping to inwardly rotate are:

- subscapularis (anterior shoulder blade muscle)
- pectoralis major
- latissimus dorsi
- teres major (greater round muscle).

The main outward rotators are:

- infraspinatus ('below-the-shoulder-blade-spine' muscle)
- teres minor (lesser round muscle).

Flexibility of upper arm inward and outward rotation can be tested in the position presented in Figure 5.21.

4. Serratus anterior (anterior serrated muscle)

(Sera = saw; ante = in front of). This muscle plays a very important role in stabilizing the shoulder. It arises from 8, 9 or even 10 ribs, and passes backwards along the rib cage and in behind the scapula (shoulder blade) to be inserted into the medial inner border of the scapula (should be assigned to group B).

Serratus anterior prevents the scapula from being pressed backwards when the body supports itself on its arms (Figure 5.22A; right upper body viewed from the side). It is trained in all types of exercises where the body is supported by the arms (Figure 5.22C).

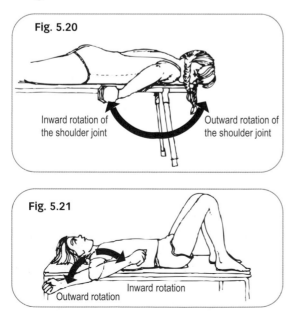

Fig. 5.20

Inward rotation of the shoulder joint

Outward rotation of the shoulder joint

Fig. 5.21

Outward rotation

Inward rotation

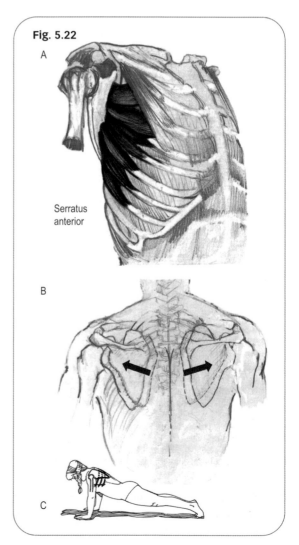

Fig. 5.22

A

Serratus anterior

B

C

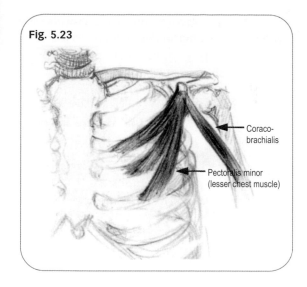

Fig. 5.23

Coraco-brachialis

Pectoralis minor (lesser chest muscle)

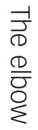

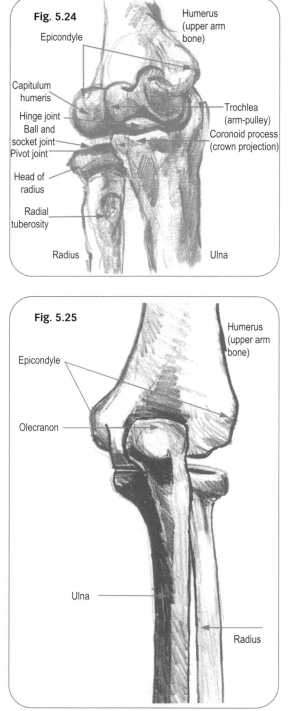

Fig. 5.24

Humerus (upper arm bone)

Epicondyle

Capitulum humeris

Hinge joint
Ball and socket joint
Pivot joint

Head of radius

Radial tuberosity

Radius

Trochlea (arm-pulley)

Coronoid process (crown projection)

Ulna

Fig. 5.25

Humerus (upper arm bone)

Epicondyle

Olecranon

Ulna

Radius

Figure 5.22B (upper body viewed from the back) shows how the scapula moves when serratus anterior contracts.

The two muscles shown in Figure 5.23 play no significant role in athletics but, nevertheless, contribute to stabilizing the scapula. Figure 5.23 (left side viewed from the front) presents the location of pectoralis minor (lesser chest muscle) and coracobrachialis.

The elbow

Elbow joint

Elbow movements occur at three separate joints: hinge joint between the humerus (upper arm bone) and ulna; pivot joint between the ulna and radius; and ball and socket joint between the humerus and the radius.

The projections and articular surfaces concerned with the function of the elbow joint can be seen in Figures 5.24 and 5.25, which respectively show the right elbow viewed from the front (with the palm of the hand facing forwards) and the right elbow viewed from the back.

- Epicondyles give attachment to the muscles which move the hand at the wrist joint.
- Radial tuberosity gives attachment to the biceps brachii (two-headed arm muscle) (see also Figure 5.26A).

- Olecranon process (elbow projection) gives attachment to triceps brachii (three-headed arm muscle) (p. 122).
- Articular surface of the humerus (upper arm bone) at its hinge joint with the elbow: the trochlea (arm-pulley).

- Articular surface of the ulna at its hinge joint with the elbow: the coronoid process = (crown projection).
- Articular surface of the ball and socket joint: the capitulum (small head).
- Head of the radius, which forms the 'socket' part of the ball and socket joint.

A relatively common difference between men and women can be seen in the olecranon process and the hollow of the humerus into which it is received when the arm is stretched.

The olecranon process and its corresponding fossa (hollow) differ in depth between men and women, rendering women more prone to over-stretch the elbow joint than men.

Elbow flexion

The three most important flexors are shown in Figure 5.26.

A. Biceps brachii (two-headed arm muscle)
B. Brachialis (upper arm muscle)
C. Brachioradialis (arm–radius muscle)

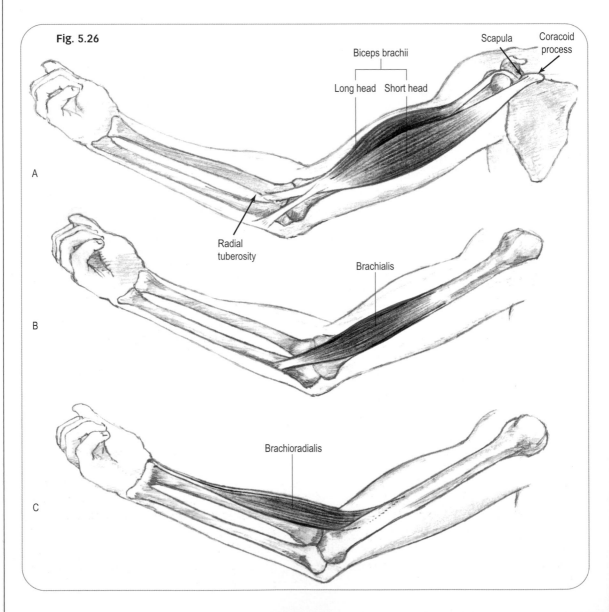

Fig. 5.26

Biceps brachii

Long head   Short head

Scapula   Coracoid process

A

Radial tuberosity

Brachialis

B

Brachioradialis

C

Origin for biceps brachii:

- Short head: the coracoid process (crow's beak projection).
- Long head: the upper rim of the scapula's (shoulder blade's) articular surface.

Insertion:

Radial tuberosity (3)(a roughened surface at the upper end of the shaft of the radius).

Function:

1. Flexes (bends) the elbow.
2. Rotates the forearm so that the palm of the hand turns upward or forwards (supination).
3. Swings the upper arm forwards (flexion of the shoulder joint).

In order to develop strength in the elbow flexors, the barbell (or whatever) must be grasped with the palms of the hands turned upwards, since this is the only way the biceps can work with maximal strength.

In Figure 5.27 the girl's hands are supinated (they grasp the bar from underneath). Therefore all her flexors work maximally.

In Figure 5.28 the boy's hands are pronated (they grasp the bar from above), which means that his biceps cannot work maximally. Instead he subjects his other flexors to a heavier work load. In general training, one should alternate between these two methods. Figure 5.29 shows arm pull-ups with (A) pronated forearm and (B) supinated forearm.

The long tendon of origin of the biceps (seen in Figures 5.26A and 5.30) passes through the shoulder joint and emerges from the joint capsule at its attachment to the humerus (upper arm bone), where it descends in the intertubercular sulcus (the biceps groove), which is

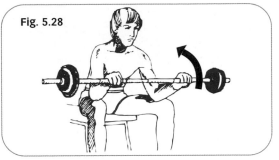

Fig. 5.28

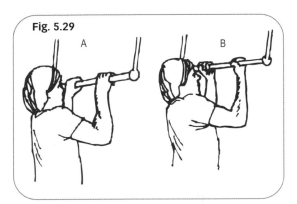

Fig. 5.29

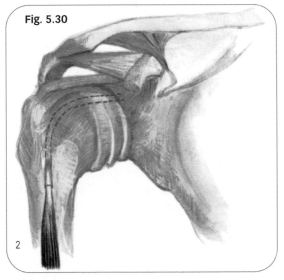

Fig. 5.30

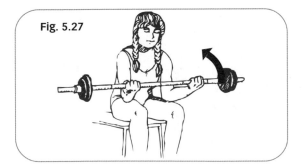

Fig. 5.27

between the anterior projection (lesser tuberosity) and the outer projection (greater tuberosity) (see Figure 5.3). Because of this, the biceps contribute greatly to the stability of the shoulder joint. A person who has dislocated his shoulder has, therefore, good reason to build up the

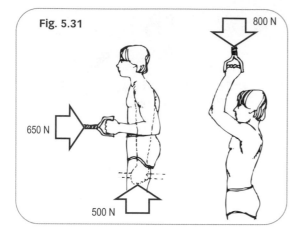

Fig. 5.31

800 N

650 N

500 N

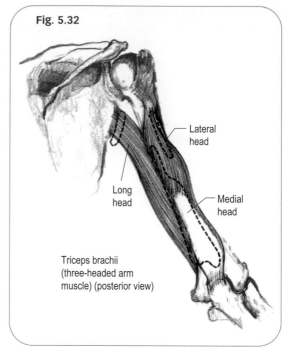

Fig. 5.32

Lateral head

Long head

Medial head

Triceps brachii
(three-headed arm
muscle) (posterior view)

strength of his biceps muscle since by doing so he may help to prevent recurrent dislocations.

Biceps strength depends, among other things, on the position of the upper arm. If we consider the distance between the origin and insertion of the biceps muscle, we see that it is greater when the arm points straight upwards than when it hangs down.

Thus, the capacity of the biceps to bend the arm with force is greater when the arm is directed upwards. The quantities in Figure 5.31 give the approximate relationship between strength to carry, pull towards the body and lift oneself up.

A reasonable conclusion we can draw from Figure 5.31 is that the human body is better suited to hang in trees than to carry buckets.

Elbow extension

The elbow extensor, triceps brachii (three-headed arm muscle) is attached to the olecranon process (elbow projection). It has three heads. One arises from the scapula (shoulder blade) and the other two from the posterior surface of the humerus (upper arm bone).

Its function is to straighten or extend the elbow and to swing the arm backwards.

A person's strength varies in different positions depending both on the length of the muscles (p. 17) and the size of the muscles lever arm to the elbow joint. Notice that the muscle is attached far back on the olecranon process in order to allow the most favourable moment arm possible in all elbow joint positions.

The extensor's lever arm is least (l_1) when the arm is fully flexed (Figure 5.33). At the same time, the force of the muscle is greatest. Strength (moment of force) is least when the joint is extended because the muscle force (F_2) is small. The strength of the muscle also depends on the way the arm is held in relation to the scapula. If the arm is stretched out in front of the body, the long head of the triceps is in a worse position (shorter distance between origin and insertion) than if the arm is held straight above the body. Figure 5.34 shows the approximate relationship between the strength of the triceps brachii in downward, forward, and upward presses.

Figure 5.35 is a cross section to show the location and size of the muscles of the right upper arm.

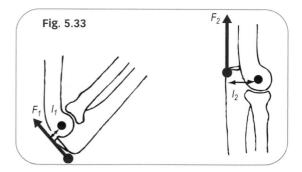

Fig. 5.33

F_2

F_1 l_1

l_2

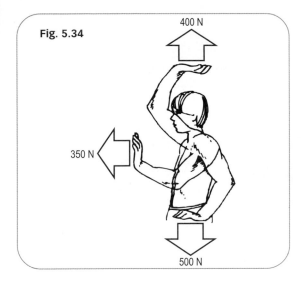

Fig. 5.34

400 N

350 N

500 N

Figure 5.36 gives suggestions for different exercises for developing strength in the triceps.

In Figures 5.37 and 5.38, you can see the relative positions between most of the muscles you have read about in this chapter so far.

Compare the elbow (Figure 5.25) with a front view of the knee joint and you will find great resemblance. When you read about flexor and extensor muscles in the elbow, compare with the corresponding muscles in the knee. The likeness gives room for lots of interesting thoughts.

Here is a list of similarities:

Olecranon process	Patella
Two joints	Two articular surfaces with meniscus
Biceps brachii	Biceps femoris
Brachialis,	Semitendinosus,
Brachioradialis	semimembranosus
Triceps long head	Rectus femoris
Triceps medial head	Vastus medialis
Triceps lateral head	Vastus lateralis

Try to find the same comparison between the shoulder and hip joints. When you find differences, try to find natural explanations.

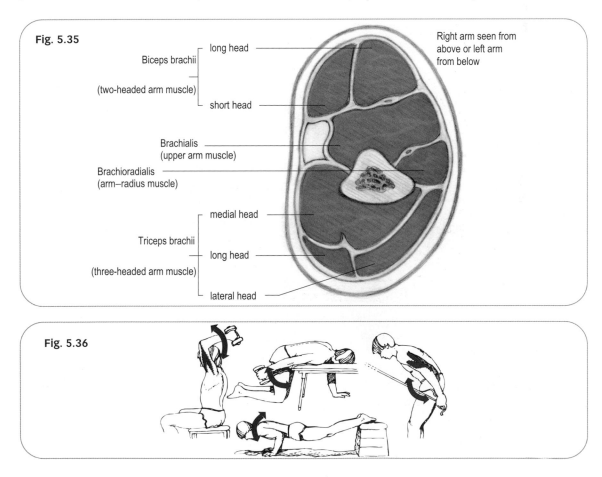

Fig. 5.35

Biceps brachii (two-headed arm muscle) — long head, short head

Right arm seen from above or left arm from below

Brachialis (upper arm muscle)

Brachioradialis (arm–radius muscle)

Triceps brachii (three-headed arm muscle) — medial head, long head, lateral head

Fig. 5.36

123

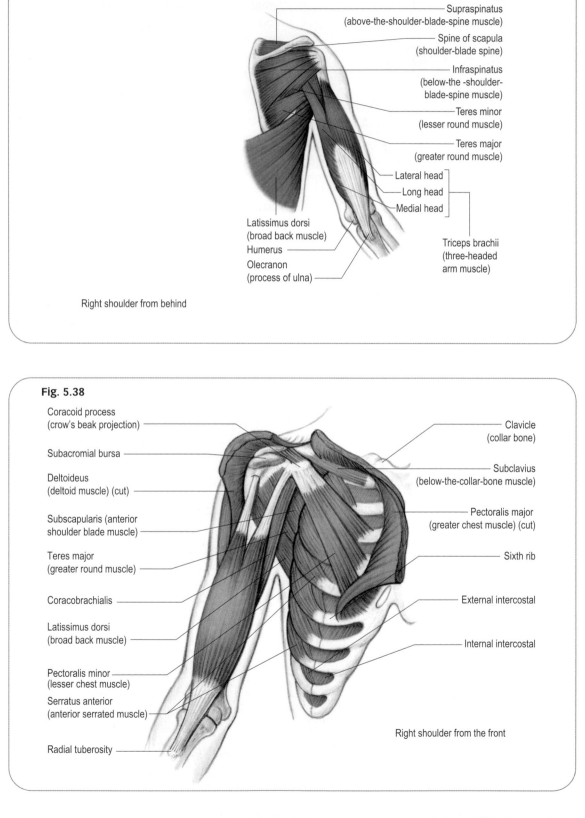

Fig. 5.37

Supraspinatus
(above-the-shoulder-blade-spine muscle)

Spine of scapula
(shoulder-blade spine)

Infraspinatus
(below-the -shoulder-
blade-spine muscle)

Teres minor
(lesser round muscle)

Teres major
(greater round muscle)

Lateral head
Long head
Medial head

Triceps brachii
(three-headed
arm muscle)

Latissimus dorsi
(broad back muscle)
Humerus
Olecranon
(process of ulna)

Right shoulder from behind

Fig. 5.38

Coracoid process
(crow's beak projection)

Subacromial bursa

Deltoideus
(deltoid muscle) (cut)

Subscapularis (anterior
shoulder blade muscle)

Teres major
(greater round muscle)

Coracobrachialis

Latissimus dorsi
(broad back muscle)

Pectoralis minor
(lesser chest muscle)

Serratus anterior
(anterior serrated muscle)

Radial tuberosity

Clavicle
(collar bone)

Subclavius
(below-the-collar-bone muscle)

Pectoralis major
(greater chest muscle) (cut)

Sixth rib

External intercostal

Internal intercostal

Right shoulder from the front

The wrist

Wrist joint

The skeleton of the hand consists of eight carpals (bones of the wrist), five metacarpals (bones of the hand) and fourteen phalanges (bones of the fingers).

The hand changes position by movement of the wrist, which is a condyloid joint. It is formed by the articulation of three of the wrist bones with the radius. Figure 5.39 shows the right hand with palm turned forwards (supinated according to Figure 5.40F).

The movements allowed at the wrist joint are (Figure 5.40):

A. flexion (palms towards you)
B. extension (palms away from you)
C. abduction (flat hand tilted outwards) and
D. adduction (flat hand tilted inwards).

The movements involved in turning the hand are called (Figure 5.40):

E. pronation and
F. supination.

Supination and pronation occur between the bones of the forearm (at the pivot joint formed by the ulna and radius, see Figure 5.24), and not at the wrist joint. The muscles that bring about rotation of the forearm, and thereby turn the hand, are called pronators and supinators. The diagrams below present the most important of these.

However, by far the strongest supinator of the hand is the biceps brachii (two-headed arm muscle) (p. 120).

The supinators are stronger (have a greater moment of force) than the pronators. This relationship has been taken into account in the manufacture of such things as screws. Thus, the thread is constructed in such a way that a right-handed person uses supinated movements to screw it into an object, and thereby allows his muscles to work concentrically. He can easily

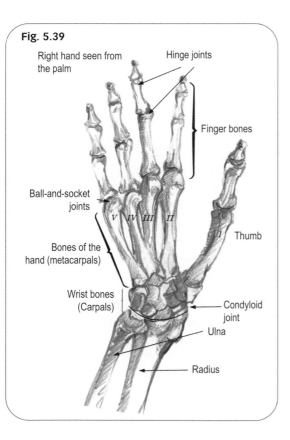

Fig. 5.39

Right hand seen from the palm

Hinge joints

Finger bones

Ball-and-socket joints

V IV III II

I Thumb

Bones of the hand (metacarpals)

Wrist bones (Carpals)

Condyloid joint

Ulna

Radius

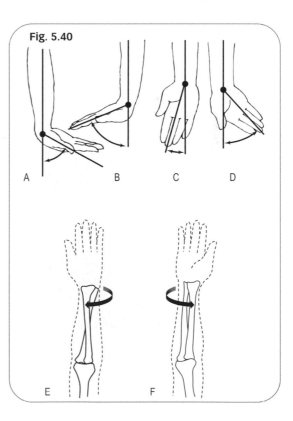

Fig. 5.40

A B C D

E F

125

feel how the biceps brachii works with great force. If the screw is so troublesome that he cannot quite manage it, he locks his wrist (lets supinators act statically (or isometrically) – see the curve on p. 21) – and thus produces rotation

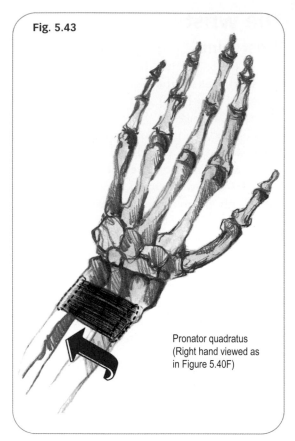

Fig. 5.43

Pronator quadratus
(Right hand viewed as
in Figure 5.40F)

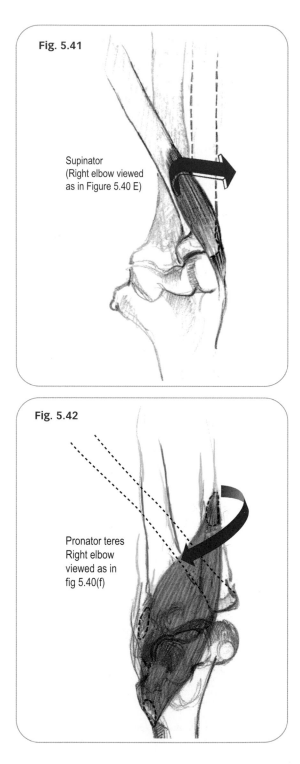

Fig. 5.41

Supinator
(Right elbow viewed
as in Figure 5.40 E)

Fig. 5.42

Pronator teres
Right elbow
viewed as in
fig 5.40(f)

by bending his elbow and rotating his shoulder joint outwards.

Of the 20 or so muscles responsible for the wrist's movements, the largest and most important are those attached to the epicondyles of the humerus (upper arm bone). The abductors and extensors of the wrist arise from the lateral (external) epicondyle.

Figure 5.44 shows some muscles (right arm viewed from the back) that are brought into action when a person hits a backhand or lifts a hammer. The term 'tennis elbow' means that the area of origin of these muscles is injured. The following can be seen in Figure 5.44:

1. Extensor digitorum (finger extensor)
2. Extensor carpi radialis (radius–wrist extensor); passes down the radius and
3. Extensor carpi ulnaris (ulna–wrist extensor); passes down the ulra.

The adductors and flexors of the wrist arise from the medial (internal) epicondyle of the humerus

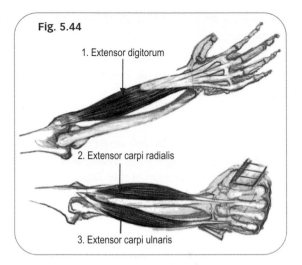

Fig. 5.44

1. Extensor digitorum
2. Extensor carpi radialis
3. Extensor carpi ulnaris

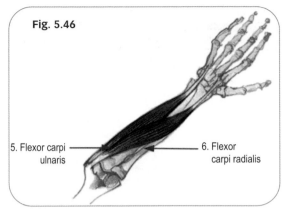

Fig. 5.46

5. Flexor carpi ulnaris
6. Flexor carpi radialis

(upper arm bone). Adduction and flexion are the movements responsible for such actions as throwing or hitting a forehand smash. Injuries caused by overexertion in these types of activities are called thrower's elbow, golfer's elbow, etc.

All the muscles in Figures 5.45 and 5.46 (right hand with the palm turned forwards) arise from the medial (internal) epicondyle of the humerus (upper arm bone):

4. Flexor digitorum (finger flexor)
5. Flexor carpi ulnaris (ulna–wrist flexor)
6. Flexor carpi radialis (radius–wrist flexor).

For the prevention of injuries such as tennis elbow, strength should be trained in moderate doses. The exercises should subject the elbow

to only light loads. They should provide both static and dynamic training. Movements should be produced in all directions allowed by the wrist. Examples of suitable loads for these exercises are dumbbells, clubs and rackets (Figures 5.47 and 5.48). Figure 5.47A and B show movements towards the thumb (abduction)

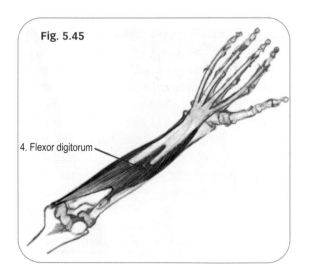

Fig. 5.45

4. Flexor digitorum

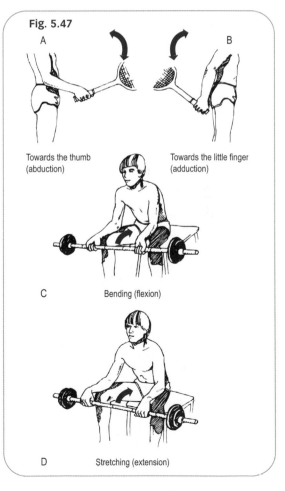

Fig. 5.47

A B

Towards the thumb (abduction)   Towards the little finger (adduction)

C   Bending (flexion)

D   Stretching (extension)

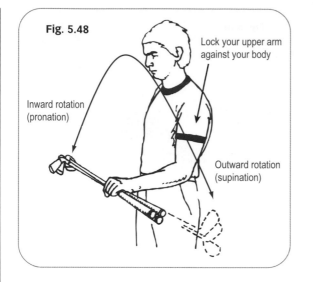

Fig. 5.48

Lock your upper arm against your body

Inward rotation (pronation)

Outward rotation (supination)

and towards the little finger (adduction) respectively. Figures 5.47C and D illustrate bending (flexion) and stretching (extension) respectively.

The following movements (Figure 5.49 A–C) can be recommended for limbering up

the wrists and, possibly, stretching the wrist muscles.

A. Lock your hands loosely and roll them around.
B. Place the palms of your hands on the ground and press lightly. Keep your arms straight. Try to hold your wrists at right angles to your arms.
C. As in B, except that you could press the back of your hand against a wall, or use your other hand as shown in the diagram.

Notice that movements involving flexion C are somewhat less flexible than those involving extension B.

When looking at strength training for shoulders and arm the discussions resemble those for the hip and knee. There are six directions of movement in the shoulder and two main movements in the elbow. The possibility to rotate much more in the forearm differs from what can be done in the knee joint. You will be using all muscles in the shoulder and upper arm if you either pull or push in different directions. The load can be your own body, handles, disc bar or different specially constructed apparatus in a gym. Remember that the weight of your body is often all you need in order to effectively strengthen the arm muscles.

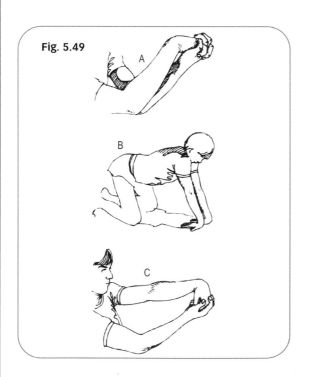

Fig. 5.49

A

B

C

Pushing

What happens if you practise in some of the positions indicated in Figure 5.50A–H? The figures in the pictures suggests how many kilos you should have, doing a bench press instead, and still experience the same stress for the muscles involved. For all variants, (bench press included), it is true that the closer your hands the more demand there is on the triceps brachii (three-headed arm muscle). The further apart the hands the more demand is put on pectoralis major and the anterior part of the deltoideus (deltoid muscle). This is because with the hands close together almost all motion takes place in the elbow and with the hands wide apart the shoulder joint comes more into action. (Try it, feel it and watch it.)

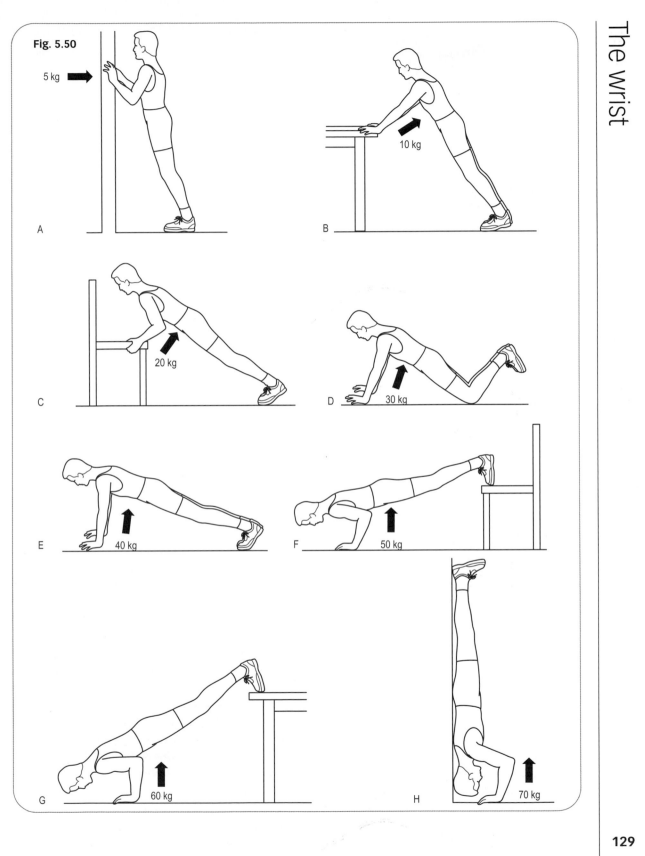

Fig. 5.50

A 5 kg

B 10 kg

C 20 kg

D 30 kg

E 40 kg

F 50 kg

G 60 kg

H 70 kg

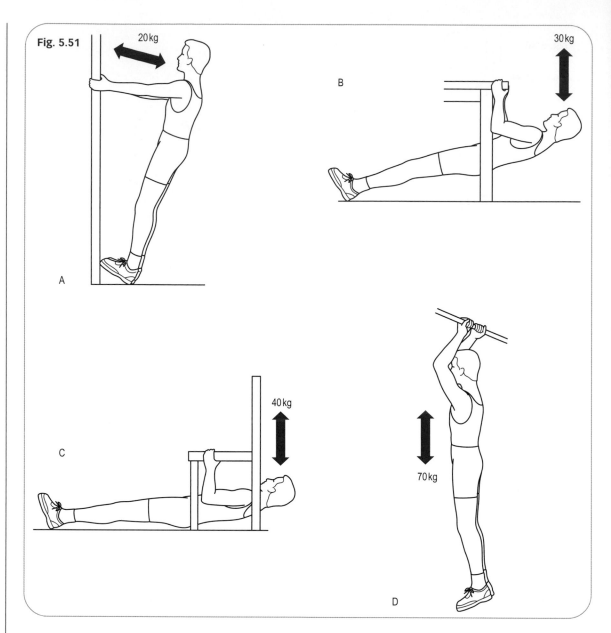

Fig. 5.51

Pulling

The same kind of discussion concerning Figure 5.50 can be conducted about Figure 5.51 A–D. The number noted in the figures is again equivalent to how many kilos you should choose on a disc bar or a pulling device.

A handle with half the load in one hand of course gives the same effect. The type of grip is of subordinate meaning when pushing but not when pulling. With 'under-grip' (as in Figure 5.52A) you stress mainly the biceps brachii (two-headed arm muscle). With 'thumbs up' (as in Figure 5.52B) you stress mainly the brachialis (upper arm muscle). With 'over-grip' (as in Figure 5.52C) you stress mainly the brachioradialis (arm–radius muscle).

The deltoideus (deltoid muscle) acts like three different muscles and should be stressed in three different directions (see Figure 5.16).

1. Backwards and up – extension.
2. Straight out – abduction.
3. Forwards and up – flexion.

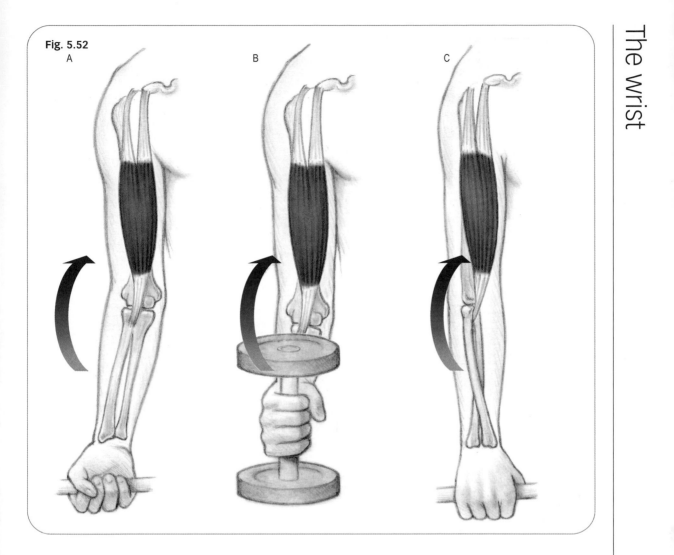

Fig. 5.52

A   B   C

The pectoralis major (greater chest muscle) also acts like three muscles (Figure 5.11) and is trained together with the deltoid muscle in the positions shown in Figure 5.53.

With pulling movements (rowing, swimming, cross country skiing, climbing …) you specially train the latissimus dorsi (broad back muscle) as well as the deltoid muscle. Figure 5.54 shows some other examples.

All movements made with effort to reach far are done by changing the position of the scapula (shoulder blade). This is mainly done by the trapezius muscle, a large muscle that will automatically be strengthened if you use exercises where the hand reaches extreme positions.

After having learned a lot about different principles concerning anatomy, training muscles for strength and flexibility you should now be prepared to choose, vary, select loads and so on in order to get good results. You should also be well prepared to give advice to others about the number of reps, set and changes in movement pattern. In the next chapter we will change focus from anatomy to biomechanics. In other words we will discuss how your muscles can handle forces from 'outside' and produce things like a javelin throw, tennis smash, football kick, high jump, somersault, pirouette and skating and so on.

If you have a triangle and you cut off one of the tips, you end up with a geometrical figure

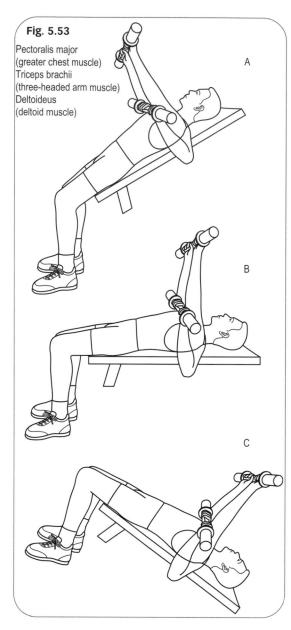

Fig. 5.53

Pectoralis major
(greater chest muscle)
Triceps brachii
(three-headed arm muscle)
Deltoideus
(deltoid muscle)

A

B

C

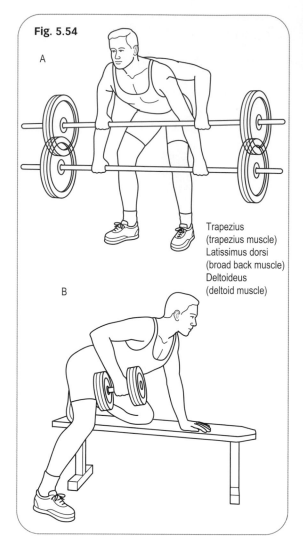

Fig. 5.54

A

Trapezius
(trapezius muscle)
Latissimus dorsi
(broad back muscle)
Deltoideus
(deltoid muscle)

B

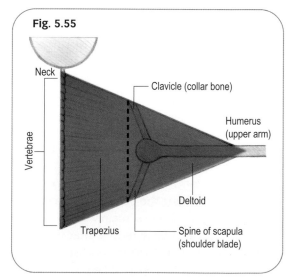

Fig. 5.55

Neck

Clavicle (collar bone)

Humerus
(upper arm)

Vertebrae

Deltoid

Trapezius

Spine of scapula
(shoulder blade)

called a trapezium and a new smaller triangle (delta) (Figure 5.55). The two large muscles covering the shoulder joint have their names from the geometrical figures mentioned above. The trapezius muscle adjusts the scapula and the deltoideus takes care of the position of the arm. They act like one single multifunctional muscle.

Chapter 6

Sports mechanics

A basic understanding of the laws of mechanics is necessary for the study of movement. When we are familiar with these laws, we can more readily analyse and design suitable exercises. Unfortunately, when athletic performance is described with the aid of the laws of mechanics, the discussion tends to be too theoretical. In this section we will consider a few concepts that are directly applicable to the practical understanding of how and why exercises are performed in a certain way.

The concepts that will be described in this chapter with diagrams as well as with formulae will be:

I. Force.
II. Centre of gravity.
III. Acceleration.
IV. Impulse and momentum.
V. Circular motion.
VI. Moment of inertia and angular momentum.

(The concept 'torque' or 'moment of force' has already been described in Chapter 2 and will be used in this chapter without further explanation).

I. Force (F)

The forces considered in this section are: force of gravity, normal force, muscle force, friction and air resistance. The muscle force is called internal force and the others are called external forces.

External forces
(a) Force of gravity (F_{mg})

The force of gravity is the mutual force of attraction between masses; it is the force that pulls an object towards the centre of the earth. The heavier the object is the larger the force of gravity will be.

Newton decided to introduce a unit of force. When this force unit acted on a mass (m) of one kilogram the velocity of the object upon which the force acted would increase by 1.0 metre per second every second. The correlation was described with the help of the expression:

$F = m \times a$ (Force = mass × acceleration)

This is sometimes called Newton's second law of motion.

This specific unit of force was later named 1 Newton (N). The expression can be described as follows: If a force of 1 N acts on a body with a mass of 1 kg the acceleration will be 1 m/s/s. Newton discovered that the gravitational pull on 1 kg is 9.81 N (on 2 kg it is 2 × 9.81 N etc). The quantity 9.81 N is the force of gravity acting on 1 kg on the surface of the earth, represented by the letter g.

A body that weighs *m* kilograms is then acted on by a force of gravity that can be written *mg* newtons.

The gravitational force acting on an object of mass $m = 5$ kg is, in other words, 5×9.81 N. The number 9.81 is often rounded off to 10. The gravitational force acting on 60 kg will consequently be 600 N. You can get an idea of how much 1 N is if you hold something in your hand that weighs 0.1 kg, since the force of gravity acting on 0.1 kg is 1 N. Figure 6.1 shows two jumping movements that are impeded by gravitational pull.

A leg weighs about 20% of total body weight. If you swing a leg forwards and upwards, 20% of the body weight will move in a circular course upwards. This makes the whole body's centre of gravity move in the same way, with a radius of arc that is 20% of the radius of the arc described by the centre of gravity of the legs.

If a person changes position from A to B in Figure 6.2 the centre of gravity (CG) will move from point 1 to 2 depending on the movement of the leg, and from point 2 to 3, depending on the movement of the arm. Since the weight of the arms is about one third that of the legs the radius of the arc described by the arm-swing will be one third of the radius of the arc described by the leg.

Suppose that a person is falling freely straight down (Figure 6.3). The centre of gravity will be moving in a straight line downwards. If the person pulls up his legs the upper body will be pulled in the opposite direction. The centre of gravity has moved slightly closer to the head but the

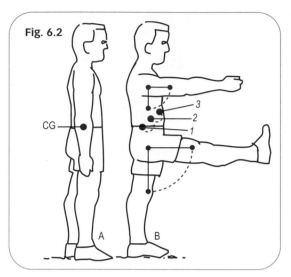

Fig. 6.2

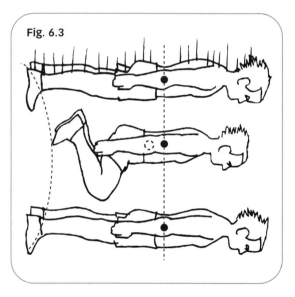

Fig. 6.3

upper body has moved as much in the other direction. The centre of gravity will still lie in the same vertical line as before. If the legs are straightened out again the head will go back to the original position. The line for the centre of gravity has not changed.

When a basketball-player wants to 'hang' in the air to get complete control of a shot, he consciously or unconsciously makes a compensating movement with his legs. In Figure 6.4 the paths of the head and the centre of gravity are drawn as broken lines. By flexing the legs at the end of the up-going phase and straightening them at the beginning of the down-going phase of the jump,

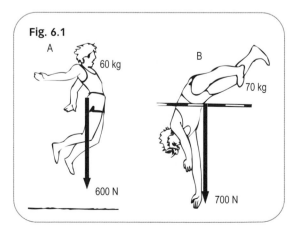

Fig. 6.1

A

60 kg

600 N

B

70 kg

700 N

Fig. 6.4

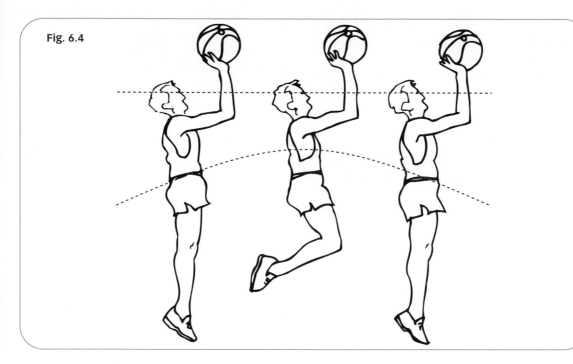

the head will be forced to follow the upper line. This pattern of movement gives the desired rigidity in the upper body during the 'shot-making' moment.

The line of the centre of gravity is decided at take-off and cannot be changed while in the air. The head's height can be regulated by changing the position of the legs or the arms (Figure 6.5).

Fig. 6.5

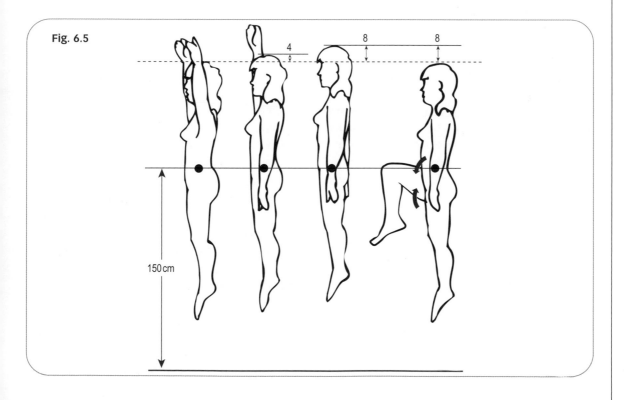

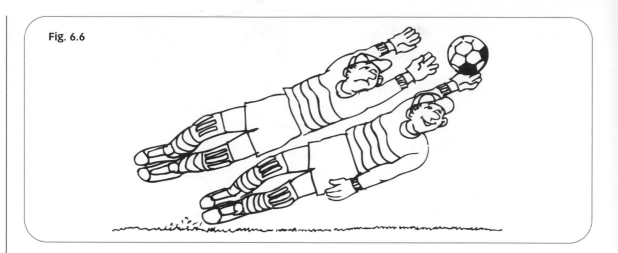

Fig. 6.6

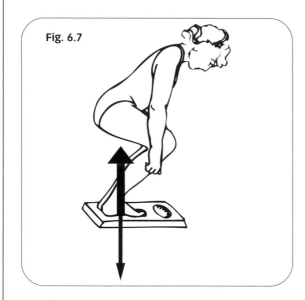

Fig. 6.7

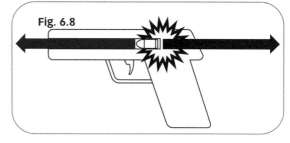

Fig. 6.8

The same rules are valid for a goalkeeper trying to reach a ball (Figure 6.6). It is possible to reach out further with one arm if the other is held in the opposite direction.

The examples above all have one thing in common, namely that a muscle pulls as much at its origin as at its insertion. This is just a special case of Newton's statement that no force acts on an object unless there is an equal force in the opposite direction acting on another object. This law is called 'the law of action–reaction forces' and reads as follows:

A force is always followed by an equal force acting in the opposite direction on another object. (This is sometimes called Newton's third law.)

The figures discussed below give examples of so-called action and reaction forces.

Example 1. In Figure 6.7, the person pushes downwards with her weight on the scale. The scale reacts by pushing upwards with a force of the same magnitude (this force is called the Normal force).

Example 2. In Figure 6.8, the gas that is produced when a gunpowder-load explodes partly pushes on the bullet (acceleration force) and partly on the pistol (recoil); the forces are equally large, but act in different directions (collinear forces) and on different objects.

Example 3. In Figure 6.9A, the skier uses his muscles and pushes the ski stick down and backwards towards the snow (a). The snow pushes back upwards-forwards with an equal force. The force on the skier will be according to the arrow (b).

When a golf club strikes a ball this pair of forces also come into operation, one acting on the ball and the other on the club (Figure 6.9B). The curves below (Figure 6.10) show how the

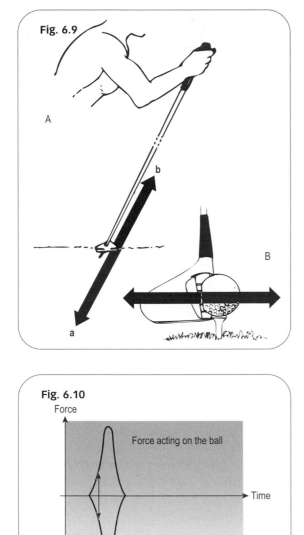

Fig. 6.9

Fig. 6.10

Force

Force acting on the ball

Time

Force acting on the club

force on the ball starts at zero, grows to a maximum and then decreases to zero again. The reaction force is exactly the same in size but is collinear.

(b) Normal force (F_N)

Normal force (force perpendicular to a surface) is exerted on a body when it comes into contact with the ground. If a person weighing 60 kg stands still on flat ground, he will be exerting a force of 600 N on the ground. The reaction force exerted on his body by the ground will also be 600 N (Figure 6.11). Thus, these two forces are equal in magnitude but act in opposite directions and on

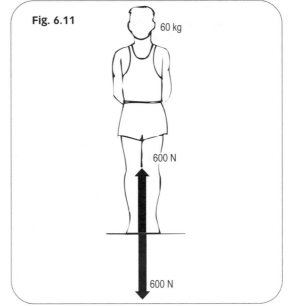

Fig. 6.11

60 kg

600 N

600 N

different objects. They constitute a so-called pair of collinear forces, where one of the forces is called 'action' and the other the 'reaction'. Some further examples of action–reaction forces are given on pp. 140–141.

The magnitude of the normal force depends on the force with which a person presses against the ground (i.e. how heavy he is) and to what extent he activates his hip, knee and ankle extensors. In taking off for a jump, swinging a leg forward while running and landing from a jump, the normal force can be as much as three to four times the body's own weight (mg) (Figure 6.12A and B).

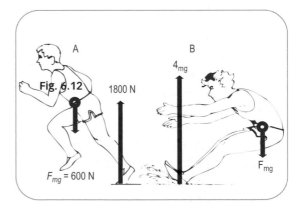

Fig. 6.12

A
B

$4mg$

1800 N

$F_{mg} = 600$ N

F_{mg}

If the person in Figure 6.13 bends her knees and then stops in a lower position the normal force varies, as shown in Figure 6.14.

As long as the person shown in Figure 6.14 is standing still, the force of gravity (F_{mg}) = normal force (F_N) but is collinear. The start of the movement downwards depends on the fact that the muscles in the legs have decreased in strength (she doesn't have the power to stand upright). The force downwards, F_{mg}, is larger than F_N. Therefore she accelerates downwards. At point 2 the acceleration is greatest. At point 3 the muscles have regained their force, so they can start braking the down-going movement. At point 4 braking is maximal. At point 5 the braking has been completed and the person is standing still again.

The curve in Figure 6.14 shows how hard the feet are pressing against the ground, an expression of normal force. It is also possible to say that the curve gives an idea of how many motor units are operating in the leg-extensor muscles during the movement.

This type of curve describes all movements that make the body's centre of gravity (CG), at a certain height above the ground, sink to a point at a lower level. Since the curve describes how hard the feet are pressing against the ground it is also possible to draw conclusions about when it is easiest to turn the feet in a new direction while doing the downward movement. At point 2 it is easiest to twist the body if you want to turn around. The quicker the downward movement, the larger the difference between F_{mg} and F_N over a short period. The lower the normal force is the easier it will be to turn skis, skates, tennis shoes etc. in a new direction. When the CG moves in the vertical plane, there will always be a period of greater freedom of movement ('relief') between the feet and the surface on which they stand. During that short time you can turn around more easily than you can when there is no vertical movement.

Temporary relief can also be gained on standing up. If you are squatting (1) and then stand up (5) the normal force will vary according to Figure 6.15 below.

If you are going to use a rising movement to relieve the pressure against the ground the relief will occur at the end of the movement (at point 4 in Figure 6.15) and not at the beginning as in a

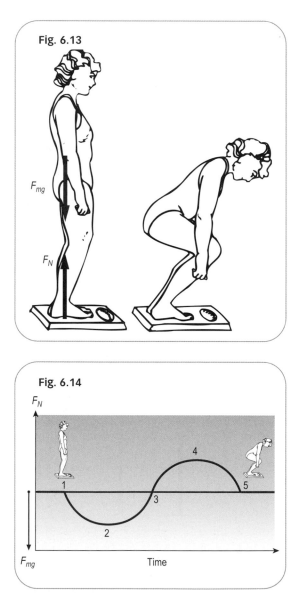

Fig. 6.13

Fig. 6.14

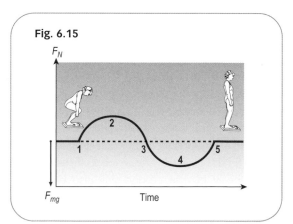

Fig. 6.15

downward movement (as seen at point 2 in Figure 6.14).

You experience the phenomena described by the curves in Figure 6.16 when you are inside an elevator. If you stood on a scale in an elevator that started to move upwards, the scale would show an increased value (point 1) when the lift started (and the floor pressed against you) and a decreased value (point 2) when it stopped (and you became lighter relative to the floor). The difference between this situation and standing up from a squatting position as in Figure 6.15 is that the elevator is moving with a constant speed for a certain time, during which the scale shows the person's real weight. If the elevator starts and moves downwards the pattern will be reversed (points 3 and 4).

Figure 6.17 shows both courses of event for an imagined movement comprising an up-going element immediately followed by a down-going element. The pressure against the ground will be almost the same as sliding the 'elevator-curves' into each other without an intervening period.

If you want to turn a pair of skis you will have double the relief period if you are moving up–down in a smooth rhythm than if you are only moving upwards. Consider how a ballerina is moving when she does repeated pirouettes or a downhill skier's moving pattern in a normal turn. An ice-hockey player uses the same method if he quickly wants to change from going forward to going backward.

If a skier moves as in Figure 6.18 the following applies. His muscles act statically as long as he skis without bending. The normal force is then 600 N if he weighs 60 kg. From points 1 to 2 he relaxes his muscles a little, with the result that less pressure is exerted on the ground (i.e. the normal force is reduced to, say, 400 N). From points 2 to 3 he halts the downward movement, which applied at point 2. He accomplishes this by working his muscles eccentrically and pressing more forcefully against the ground. From points 3 to 4 his muscles work concentrically, and they still press forcefully against the ground (max 800 N according to our example). At point 4 the skier has such upward acceleration that he reaches point 5 without pressing against the ground especially hard. He can even enjoy a moment's relaxation (400 N work load). From point 5 onwards, he stands still again and his load will once again be 600 N because his muscles act statically.

The pressure against the ground can be measured with so-called force platforms that measure the vertical force (the normal force) as well as the side forces (force of friction). In Figure 6.19, the plots in the graph show how the pressure against the ground varies when you are walking or running.

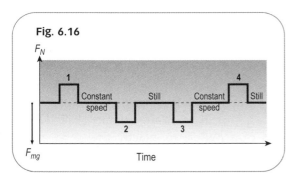

Fig. 6.16

F_N

1   Constant speed   Still   Constant speed   Still   4

2   3

F_{mg} Time

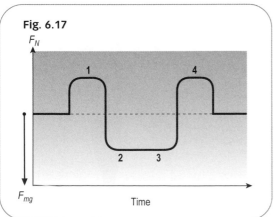

Fig. 6.17

F_N

1   4

2   3

F_{mg} Time

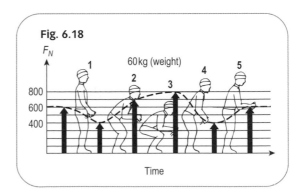

Fig. 6.18

F_N

60 kg (weight)

1   2   3   4   5

800
600
400

Time

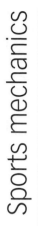

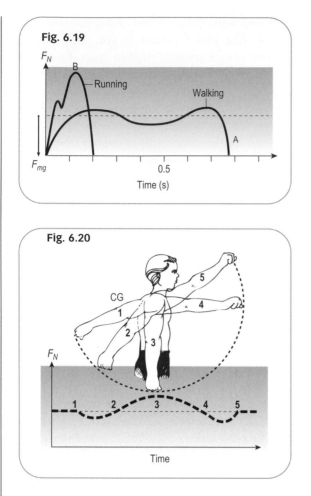

Fig. 6.19

Fig. 6.20

The normal force is also changed when a person swings his arms (Figure 6.20). Arm movements serve to both burden and unburden the body during different activities.

To be able to understand the arm's influence relative to the ground you will have to decide how the arm's CG is moving vertically. In Figure 6.20 the CG of the arms accelerates downwards between points 1 and 2, which gives a 'relief' (less force pushing against the ground). The movement in points 2 and 3 is a retardation towards the ground (the arms are moving further and further forwards and less downwards), which generates increased normal force. Points 3–4 of the figure show an acceleration upwards which gives an increased normal force; points 4–5 represent a halting period, which again decreases the normal force. The forces generated during the period covered by points 2–4 are made use of by, for example, triple jumpers, who thereby force their legs to

work maximally. This also helps the springboard diver to press down on the springboard.

In general, it can be said that a force is needed to change the velocity of a moving arm. The origin and insertion of the arm muscles are then acted upon by equal but opposing forces (i.e. the arm and the body are affected in different directions; see Figure 6.21).

When the arm is accelerated or halted by, say, the pectoralis major (greater chest muscle) or the latissimus dorsi (broad back muscle), the body is affected in the opposite direction. The arrows in Figure 6.22A–D show how the body is affected when the velocity of the arm changes. The black arrow represents the force acting on the arm and the red arrow represents the force acting on the trunk. The magnitude of the force is the same at the origin of a muscle as it is at its insertion.

If the arm:
moves backwards but is halted (A),
accelerates backwards (B),
accelerates forwards (C)
or moves forwards but is halted (D)

then the body will be affected as shown by the red arrows.

(c) Muscle forces (F_M)

Muscle forces could be called internal forces. In order to resist the forces of gravity, or to increase the normal force, the body uses muscle forces. Muscle forces affect the origin and insertion of a muscle to exactly the same extent

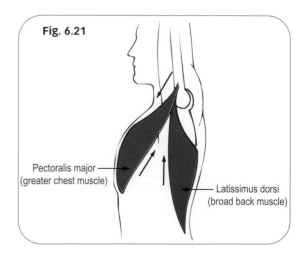

Fig. 6.21

Pectoralis major (greater chest muscle)

Latissimus dorsi (broad back muscle)

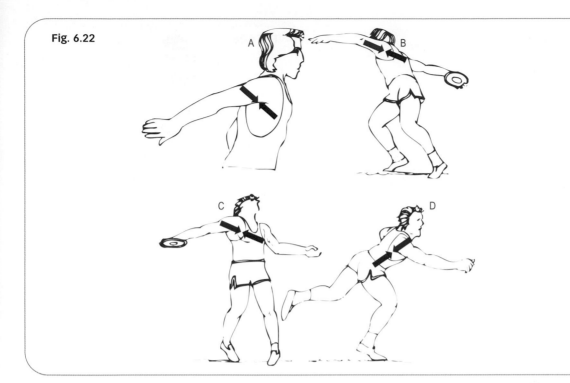

Fig. 6.22

(Figure 6.23), i.e. with equal but opposing forces. The size and structure (position of the centre of gravity) of the body parts A and B are the factors that determine what happens. Also important is whether A and B are free to move, or whether one of them is in some way 'fixed'.

Example 1. (Figure 6.23). If A and B are identical and both are free to move, they will come together much like a folding jack-knife. This is roughly what happens when a person jumps up with a straight back and flexes his hip joint. The iliopsoas muscle pulls his legs up and his trunk down. His legs are a little lighter than his trunk so they travel a longer distance as shown in Figure 6.24. It is impossible to move the legs alone.

Example 2. (Figure 6.24). If the weight of the parts differ, the lighter of the two moves the farthest.

Example 3. (Figure 6.25). If B is held stationary, only A will move.

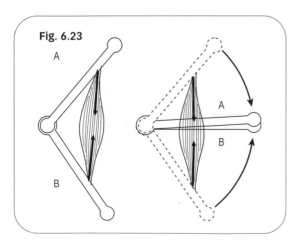

Fig. 6.23

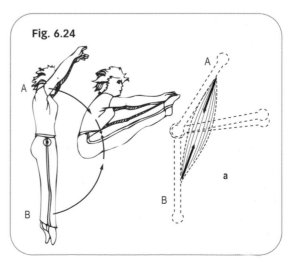

Fig. 6.24

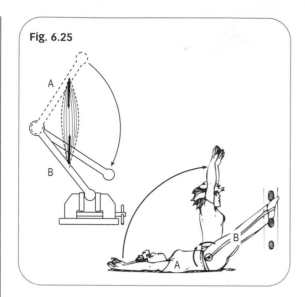

Fig. 6.25

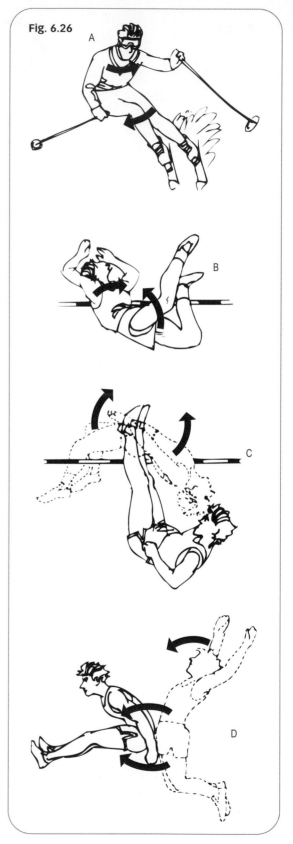

Fig. 6.26

Figure 6.26 presents different situations where both parts rotate in opposition to each other at a joint.

In Figure 6.26A, if the trunk is rotated in one direction, the skis try to turn in the opposite direction.

In pole-vaulting B, the upper part of the body is lifted over the bar by extending the hip joint and kicking backwards with the legs.

To avoid knocking the bar off with the legs in the flop style high-jump C, the hip joint is powerfully flexed once the legs have passed over the bar. By rotating the legs backwards as far as possible, the high jumper prevents the upper part of his body from rotating and avoids landing on his neck.

By thrusting his trunk forwards and continuing the rotation of his arms, the long-jumper D causes an opposite swinging movement of his legs in the landing phase of the jump.

Tendon and ligament forces. These are passive internal forces. They are brought about by muscle or external forces, i.e. the tendons and ligaments cannot themselves produce force. When subjected to severe stress from without, a ligament may rupture (Figure 6.27).

(d) Force of friction (F_μ)

Force of friction is another force that requires consideration when analysing and understanding the performance of sports. The force of

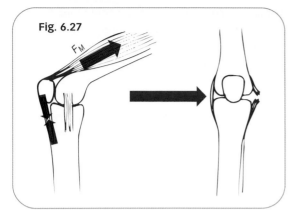

Fig. 6.27

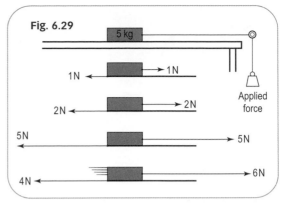

Fig. 6.29

friction is the resistance to motion of two moving objects with surfaces that touch. Every surface has minute irregularities, although some might seem even. These irregularities get hooked into each other and prevent the two different surfaces from sliding over each other (Figure 6.28).

The magnitude of the force of friction depends on the kind of materials in contact with each other (the roughness of their surfaces, the friction force μ) and how hard the two surfaces are pressed together (in other words how large the normal force (F_N) is). The magnitude of the force of friction is given by the expression:

$$F_\mu = F_N \times \mu$$

(μ is called the coefficient of friction.)

Imagine that you are about to push or pull a box along a table (Figure 6.29). Before you start, F_{mg} and F_N are acting on the box and they balance each other. When you pull with a force F and the box doesn't move, this is because the force of friction F_μ is as large as the pulling force. At a certain value of F (5 N), the box will move. The force that it takes to move the box is called fully developed friction. If you act on the box with more force there will be a surplus of force and the box will accelerate to the right.

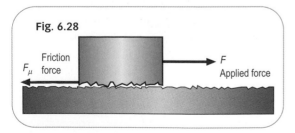

Fig. 6.28

Friction
F_μ force

F
Applied force

Suppose that the box on the table in Figure 6.29 weighs 5.0 kg; the normal force is 50 N. If you place 0.1 kg in a box, a pulling force of 1 N will not be sufficient to generate any movement. This is because the force of friction is also 1 N. The small irregularities on the surface of the table have hooked into irregularities on the surface of the box and hold it back with a restraining force of 1 N. At a load of 2 N the same thing happens: the box does not move. At a pulling force of 5 N the edge of the irregularities that are restraining the box loses its grip. The coefficient of friction between the two surfaces is in this case established to be 0.1 (5 N/50 N = 0.1).

If you pull with a force in excess of 5 N there will be a surplus of force, which makes the box accelerate. (As indicated in Figure 6.31, the box has less resistance from irregularities when it moves than when it stands still).

Coefficients of friction usually have values between 0 and 1. If the coefficient of friction is more than 1 it will take more force to push or drag the object along the surface than to lift it and carry it away. The friction existing between two cartilage surfaces lubricated with synovial fluid is among the lowest known. Between snow and a well waxed ski the coefficient of friction can be as low as 0.04. Between a skating blade and ice the coefficient of friction is around 0.01. High forces of friction are required between, for example, car tyres and the road surface. Excessively high forces of friction between sole and floor can easily cause sprains. Here, a short low-resistance 'gliding phase' is aimed for, so that the leg and foot muscles will have time to adapt to the load and thereby have time to stabilize the foot joint.

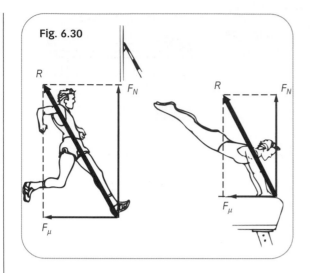

Fig. 6.30

In Figure 6.30 the force of friction of the foot and the hands are diagramatically illustrated in two different situations. The normal forces are also drawn out in the figure. F_N and F_μ are then summated giving the result R. In both cases R can be called thrust.

The graph shown in Figure 6.31 shows what happens when a body lying on the ground is acted on with greater and greater force parallel to the ground. At a low force the force of friction manages to hold the object back in place. The force of friction has the same value as the applied force and so the object stays still. At a certain point the applied force will make the object move and slide away. This value of the force of friction is called fully developed (static)

friction. When the object has developed a certain amount of speed, the force of friction will lessen slightly; and at this point dynamic friction comes into play.

Frictional forces behave differently for wet and dry surfaces. We talk about wet friction and dry friction. Examples of wet friction are a skating blade moving over ice and a ski moving over snow.

As already mentioned, the reason why fully developed (static) friction is greater than dynamic friction is that when the object is standing still the irregularities in the contacting surfaces sink deeper down into each other than when the surfaces slide over each other. This can be seen when a car brakes. If the tyres become locked, causing a gliding movement (dynamic friction), the braking force will be less than when the tyres are rolling. When a tyre is rolling, every point on the surface of the tyre that comes into contact with the road surface interlinks and the braking force can generate fully developed friction. So-called non-locking brakes prevent many accidents. In cross-country skiing (the classical style) the skier can shoot away only after the skis have come to a halt briefly. If the skis stop moving the irregularities in the contacting surfaces have time to sink into each other and there is better grip between ski and snow. The competitive skier makes this short pause, without losing too much speed, through making a small knee extension at the very end of the gliding phase, before shooting away. When you ski in the new style – 'skating' – the wax used should generate as little friction as possible. The thrust towards the ski can be achieved when the ski is still gliding, but to generate force you have to push perpendicularly towards the ski's direction of movement. This means that only part of the thrust is directed forwards, as seen in Figure 6.32. The speed therefore increases in skating since the push can happen at any speed, while in the classical style of skiing the push can not be done until the ski has come to a stop. The only difference between ice-skating and 'skating on skis' is that the friction between the ice-skating blade and the ice is remarkably lower than the friction between the ski and the snow, irrespective of

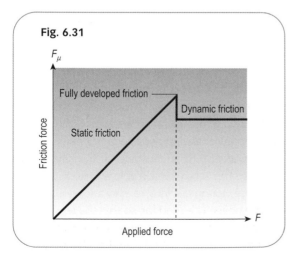

Fig. 6.31

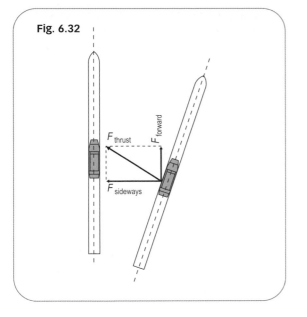

Fig. 6.32

F_{thrust}
$F_{forward}$
$F_{sideways}$

ground (F_v), and one, directed backwards, wants to throw the gravel backwards (F_h). The reaction forces countering these forces are the forces acting on the runner. These reaction forces are the normal force, F_N, and the friction force, F_μ.

The force of friction accelerates the runner forwards. Without friction you won't be moving at all. The normal force (F_N) tries to lift the runner upwards.

If $F_N > F_{mg}$ CG will accelerate upwards.
If $F_N = F_{mg}$ CG's speed won't change.
If $F_N < F_{mg}$ CG will accelerate downwards.

Figure 6.34 shows the forces that come into play when a person pulls an object. The law of action and reaction is always valid. There can be no force without another force in a collinear direction towards another object. The red forces act on the person's hands and feet. The black forces act on the handle and ground.

how good the waxing is. Not much speed is lost during the gliding phase in ordinary ice-skating.

The force that prevents even higher speed being gained is air resistance.

When running, the foot pushes against the ground with a force (F) directed slantingly backwards and downwards (Figure 6.33). This force can be divided into two components. One, directed downwards, wants to make a hole in the

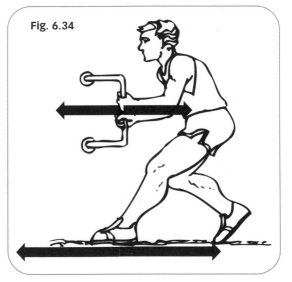

Fig. 6.34

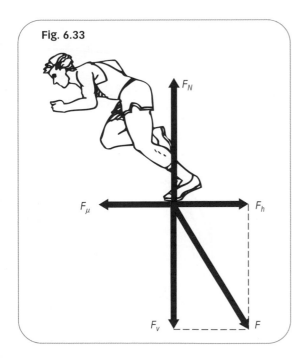

Fig. 6.33

F_N
F_μ
F_h
F_v
F

(e) Air resistance (F_a)

Air resistance met by a body that is moving in the air is caused by collision of the body with the air molecules in front of it. The molecules gain speed (gain energy) and the body loses speed (loses the same amount of energy). It can be said that the body is acted on by a braking force, which is called air resistance.

Figure 6.35 shows a parachute jumper who has just jumped out of a plane. On the left, he has not

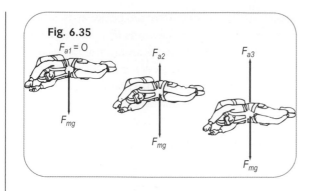

Fig. 6.35

$F_{a1} = 0$ F_{a2} F_{a3}

F_{mg} F_{mg} F_{mg}

yet developed any downward speed and therefore does not collide with any molecules: the air resistance is zero. He is acted on by the force of gravity, which makes him accelerate downwards. After some time he has reached a certain speed and pushes away a large number of air molecules, which means that besides the force of gravity, F_{mg}, he is acted on by the force of air resistance, F_{a2}, which makes the total force on the jumper, $F_{mg} - F_{a2}$. This results in lower acceleration.

The total force on the jumper would decrease with increased speed and air resistance (Figure 6.36). Since the air resistance is collinear to the force of gravity every addition of F_a will decrease the total force by the same amount. At the beginning of the jump (1) $F_{a1} = 0$ and the jumper is acted on only by the force of gravity. At (2) the air resistance has reached one-third of F_{mg} and the total force on the jumper is two-thirds of F_{mg}. At (3) the air resistance has reached its maximum; $F_{a3} = F_{mg}$, which means that $F_{total} = 0$ and no more acceleration takes place. The parachute jumper is falling at constant speed.

During a free fall from a plane a parachute jumper with a closed parachute will have reached maximal speed after about 10 seconds. The speed will cease to increase when F_{mg} and F_a are the same. The maximal speed lies somewhere between 200 and 300 km/h depending on what position the jumper adopts. Different positions give different air resistance, and thereby different maximal speeds.

In Figure 6.37 it can be seen that the area that a skier exposes when moving forwards can vary. The air resistance acting against a body depends on the size of the surface area (A) that meets the air (or being met by the air) and its velocity (v). The air resistance is proportionate to the velocity squared (v^2). A third factor is the shape of the body. The more streamlined a body is the easier it moves in the air. This is taken into consideration by giving every differently shaped body a coefficient (c), which determines the final value of the air resistance. The magnitude of the air resistance is calculated using the expression:

$$F_a = A \times v^2 \times c.$$

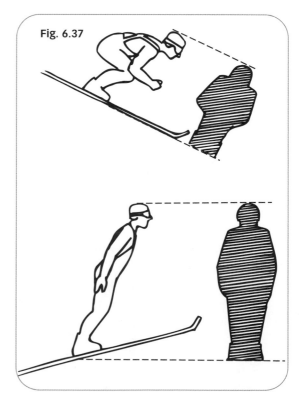

Fig. 6.37

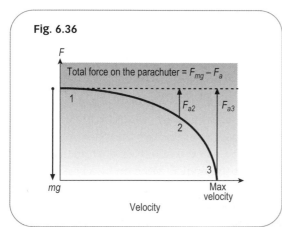

Fig. 6.36

Total force on the parachuter = $F_{mg} - F_a$

1

F_{a2} F_{a3}

2

3

F

mg

Max velocity

Velocity

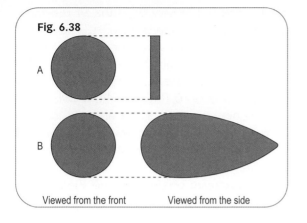

Fig. 6.38

A

B

Viewed from the front   Viewed from the side

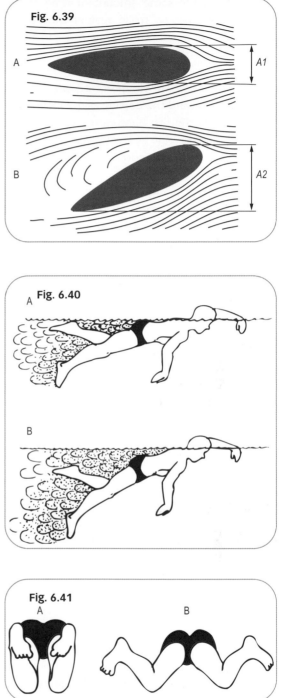

Fig. 6.39

A

A1

B

A2

Fig. 6.40

A

B

Fig. 6.41

A   B

The bodies in Figure 6.38 have the same area when viewed from the front. Viewed from the side they look completely different and have completely different streamlining coefficients. For the 'rain drop', c has a small value, which gives a low air resistance compared with that for the other body.

A change of body position often leads to a change in both A and c. The equation of air resistance has been established by experiment:

$$F_a = A \times v^2 \times c.$$

Thus, if the area is doubled, the force of resistance will be doubled, doubling the velocity gives four times the force of resistance and improving the streamlining reduces the coefficient (c), i.e. reduces air resistance. The aim in such sports as long jumping, ski jumping, skating and, in particular, downhill skiing, is to reduce air resistance. Similar considerations apply in water, but the coefficients (c) are always much greater. Therefore, in swimming, it is especially important to reduce water resistance.

Both the area and the streamline form are greater in A than in B in Figures 6.39 and 6.40.

The breaststroke kick asumes little area (A) when the heels are drawn in towards the buttocks, whereas a large area is presented when the legs kick backwards (Figure 6.41).

If an object is passed by an airstream that moves with the same speed over all sides of the object, the pressure (force/area) is the same on all sides and the object will move in a straight line. If, on the other hand, an object is shaped such that the airstream on one side is forced to take a longer route, a lower pressure will develop on that side compared to the other side. The air molecules move faster and more in parallel to the surface in order to arrive behind the object at the same time as the molecules on the other side. The faster molecules

147

do not have the same amount of time as the slower molecules to strike against the object. The slower molecules move in a more irregular path, which means that they bounce against the object more often. The more bounces the more pressure. A lower pressure on the fast side will occur and the object will be inclined to turn towards the fast airstream. A wing and a roof are objects that generate fast airstreams, producing under-pressure (F_u) on one side (Figure 6.42).

If you put a ping-pong ball in an airstream from a hairdryer, as depicted in Figure 6.43, the principle described above can be tested out very simply. The ball will stay in the stream even if it is directed at the side. The three forces acting

are the force of gravity (F_{mg}) the air resistance (F_a) and the under-pressure (F_u). The sum of these forces equals zero and the ball 'hangs miraculously' in the air.

When a ball is moving forwards at the same time as it is rotating (Figure 6.44) it will, due to friction between its surface and the air molecules, draw a part of the airstream to one side that would otherwise have flowed past on the opposite side.

The airstream on one side will thereby flow more quickly since it has to travel a longer distance in the same amount of time. A lower pressure will develop and the ball will be sucked into the faster air-stream. The ball will start to change direction.

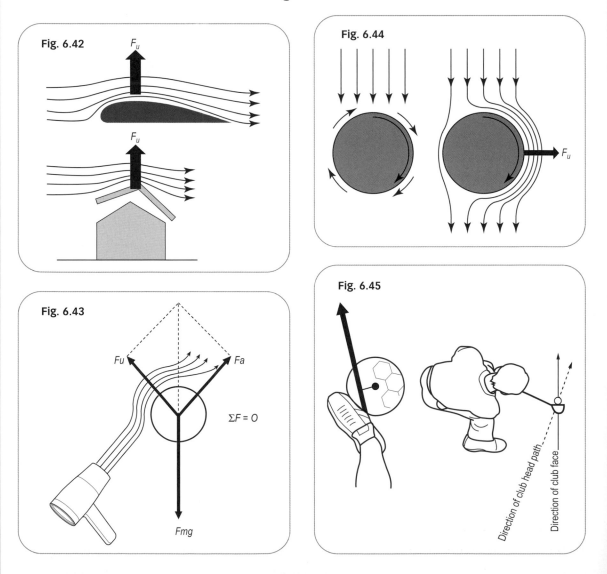

Fig. 6.42

Fig. 6.44

Fig. 6.43

$\Sigma F = 0$

Fig. 6.45

Direction of club head path

Direction of club face

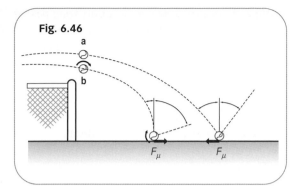

Fig. 6.46

Figure 6.45 shows how you can produce rotation while kicking or striking a ball. The football will rotate clockwise and the golf ball anticlockwise.

Figure 6.46 shows how a tennis ball with topspin (b) moves in the air and how it bounces compared to a ball with no spin at all (a).

When a ball with no spin bounces against the ground the ball is acted on by a force of friction and a normal force. If the ball has a topspin the force of friction will decrease the more the ball rotates. At a very high rotation speed the surface of the ball that touches the ground will move backwards relative to the ground. The consequence of this will be that the force of friction will decrease when the amount of topspin increases, and with very high values of the topspin the friction vector will turn and be directed forwards.

This force accelerates the ball at the bounce and the ball will therefore have a higher speed after bouncing than before. The result will be a flat, fast ball that is difficult for the opponent to control.

Rules for vectors

When we explained how the thrust in, for example, skiing depended on the fact that the force of friction and the normal force co-operated, a rule on how forces are summated was used. We will see here some examples on how to summate forces. We will also see how to divide a force into components to be able further to understand the function of a force.

Forces have <u>vector characteristics</u>. This means that they have <u>magnitude and direction</u>. Other physical quantities such as velocity, acceleration, impulse and spin are also vectors. There are also quantities that differ from vectors since they have magnitude and no direction. They are called scalars. Examples of scalars are mass, volume, temperature, time and length. Vectors can be added, subtracted, and divided into different components, according to certain rules that will be presented below.

Addition of two vectors

If two forces act at the same point and pull in the same direction (Figure 6.47A) the resultant will be oriented in the same direction with a magnitude that is equal to the sum of the forces. If the forces pull in different directions the result will be as shown in Figure 6.47B below. If the forces create an angle between them they are added as shown in Figure 6.48.

The sum of two vectors that create an angle between them is called a resultant. The parallelogram method is used to make the summation.

Since we are only interested in principles and not the precise results it is sufficient to draw the

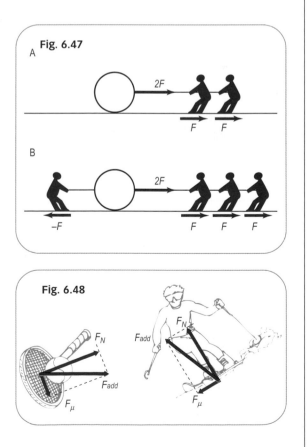

Fig. 6.47

Fig. 6.48

forces present, according to scale, as far as is possible so that we can measure the result directly from the figure. This is called graphical problem solving.

Figure 6.49 shows how two different forces that are acting on a boat crossing a river can be summated. The arrows indicate the force from the engine of the boat and the force from the water coming from the left. If you steer straight forwards the boat will travel slightly to the right. To be able to go straight forwards you will have to steer to the left so that the summated forces give a resultant oriented in the desired direction.

A vector can be moved along its own direction line without changing its result. A table can be moved either by pushing with a given force according to arrow F_1 or by pulling the table in front of oneself according to arrow F_2. The result will be the same (Figure 6.50).

All four forces in Figure 6.50 have the same magnitude.

Both F_1 and F_2 have a direction that passes through the centre of gravity of the table and both of them will move the table to the right without rotating it. Both forces act in exactly the same way on the table.

F_3 and F_4 both want to move the table but they also want to rotate it anticlockwise. There are no differences between the effects of these two forces.

The example below utilizes some of the information that we have encountered up to now.

The force of gravity F_{mg} as seen in Figure 6.51 can be moved down its line of action so that the distance to the hip joint can be compared to the distance between the pulling force of the abduction muscles on the joint. If the distances are 3:1 the muscle force F_M has to produce $3 \times F_{mg} = 1800$ N (if $F_{mg} = 600$ N) to control the motion in the hip joint. If F_{mg} and F_M are moved along their lines of force they meet at point A. They can now be added and the total force is directed straight through the head of the femur (thigh

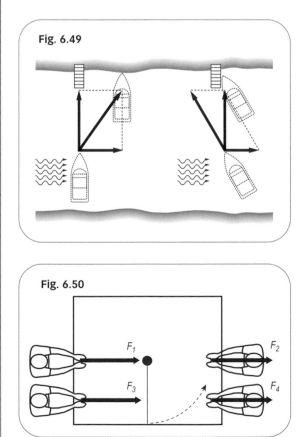

Fig. 6.49

Fig. 6.50

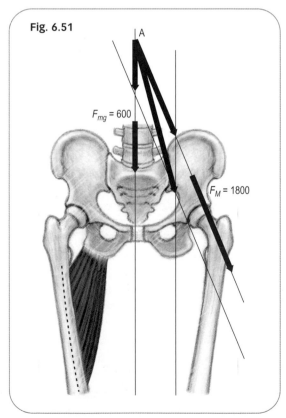

Fig. 6.51

$F_{mg} = 600$

$F_M = 1800$

bone) and along the line of the neck of the femur. The design of the slanting neck of the femur is perfectly adapted to handle the forces acting during upright walking.

Dividing a vector into components

To make it easier to determine what is happening during the execution of a movement, a force or a speed can, in some cases, be divided into components. Take the shot-put as an example. Suppose that the shot leaves the hand with a speed of 10 m/s in the direction indicated in Figure 6.52.

To determine how fast the shot is moving (a) parallel to the ground and (b) straight up in the air, at the moment of release, you divide the vector into components in these desired directions. The procedure is opposite to the one used in the parallelogram method discussed above. A parallelogram is drawn where the original vector becomes diagonal and the sides indicate the answers to the questions.

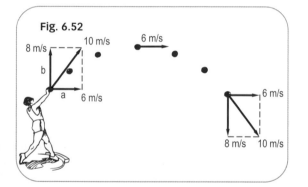

Fig. 6.52

Measuring the lengths of the arrows, (a) is 6 m/s and (b) is 8 m/s in the example above.

Now you can look at the horizontal speed by itself and consider what happens to it while the shot is in the air. Since the air resistance is almost non-existent relative to the momentum of the shot, it is possible to say that the forward speed is 6.0 m/s during the whole flight.

In the same way, you can observe the speed upwards and consider how the force of gravity first decreases this speed and thereafter increases it in the opposite direction.

When you are looking at the shot passing downwards at the same height as the point of release you will find that:

- The horizontal speed is still 6 m/s.
- The vertical speed is again 8 m/s but now directed downwards.
- The total speed is once again 10 m/s.

When using the ski-sticks shown in Figure 6.53, the skier will move in the direction in which the ski-stick is pointing.

If this force is divided into two components F_h and F_v, F_h describes the part of the thrust that accelerates the skier forward while F_v describes the part of the thrust that is directed straight upwards, easing the pressure on the ground and thereby decreasing the normal force by the same magnitude. The end-point of thrusting forward using the ski-stick provides the greater part of the acceleration gained (for a given force), although

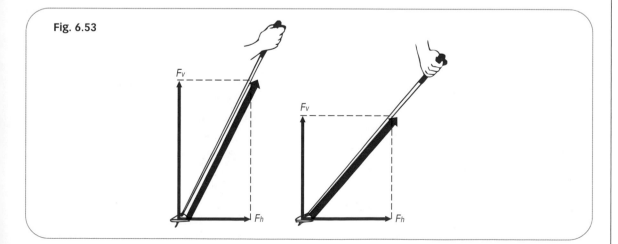

Fig. 6.53

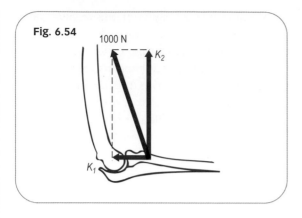

Fig. 6.54

the skier is much stronger at the beginning of the movement and creates more force at that point.

In Figure 6.54 the force with which the biceps brachii muscle (two-headed arm muscle) pulls at its insertion on the forearm is illustrated. Suppose that the force is 1000 N. How great is the force that pulls the forearm against the joint centre?

To be able to answer this question you will have to divide the force into two components, one (K_1) that is oriented in the required direction (in other words towards the centre of the elbow joint) and one (K_2) that is orientated at right angles to this line of direction. The latter component will be the one that rotates the forearm around the joint.

From the construction lines you can see how to derive the relative magnitudes of K_1 and K_2.

Figure 6.55 shows a knee in two different positions. The force from the quadriceps femoris (four-headed thigh muscle) is 1000 N in both cases.

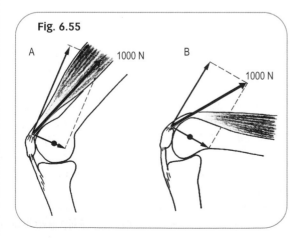

Fig. 6.55

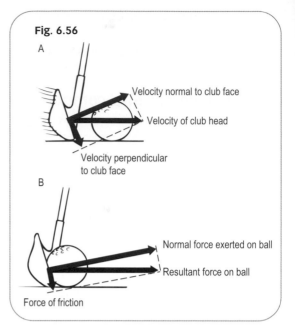

Fig. 6.56

Figure 6.55B shows how the force directed towards the centre of the joint and the part that rotates is constructed. The more the knees are bent the larger is the pressure between patella (kneecap) and femur (thigh bone).

Figure 6.56A shows a golf club that is moving straight forward in the horizontal plane. Despite this, the speed can still be divided into two imagined components, one perpendicular to the club face, which gives rise to a force on the ball as shown in Figure 6.56A, and one parallel to the club face, which creates a force of friction on the ball as shown in Figure 6.56B. The total force on the ball shows that the ball leaves the club face at an angle lower than that at which the club face is orientated.

The backspin generated will give rise to a lower pressure above the ball compared to below. This will force the ball to continue to rise in a trajectory that is steeper than the initial incline of the club face.

II. Centre of gravity

The centre of gravity (CG) of a body is the point at which it could, in theory, be suspended and remain in equilibrium regardless of its position (Figure 6.57).

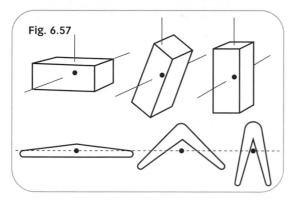

Fig. 6.57

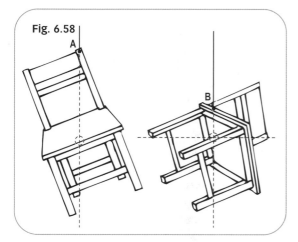

Fig. 6.58

A

B

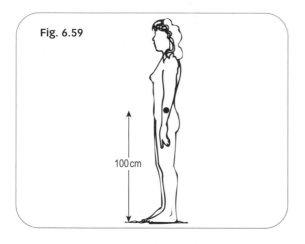

Fig. 6.59

100 cm

It is easy to find the CG in a symmetrical body; it is more difficult to do so in an asymmetrical one. Nevertheless, a trainer should be able to discern just where the CG of an athlete's body lies in any given situation. By doing so, he can correctly instruct an athlete on how to execute exercises.

The CG of a rigid body can be determined by experiment in the following way (Figure 6.58): hang the body freely at an arbitrary point A. The CG will lie on the vertical line passing through A. Hanging the body from some other point, B, gives another straight line on which the CG lies. Clearly, the CG is the intersection of the two lines.

The CG of a human body standing in the anatomical position (Figure 6.59), lies approximately in line with the navel a few centimetres in front of the third lumbar vertebra. Naturally, the location of the CG changes with changes in body position (e.g. when an arm or leg is raised).

Figure 6.60 demonstrates how the CG varies in relation to the ground. If the CG in Figure 6.59 lies 100 cm above the ground it will rise about 4 cm when an arm is raised, 8 cm when both arms are raised, 8 cm if the person lifts up the knee (see also Figure 6.60).

If a person jumps up so that her CG reaches a point 150 cm above the ground (Figure 6.61), a change in body position will not affect the height of the CG in relation to the ground. Once the body has left the ground its position on the way up will not affect the maximal height of the CG.

Although the CG reaches the same height in all four jumps as seen in Figure 6.61, the height of the hand and head above the ground varies with the final position. If both arms are lowered, the body is raised 8 cm. If one leg is raised, the rest of the body will be lowered 8 cm. The explanation for this is quite simply that the muscle groups that lift the leg (e.g. iliopsoas) affect the rest of the body with an equal but opposing force, i.e. one that pulls the body down. This also happens with the arm.

The pattern of movement in such activities as the jump shot in handball, shooting in basketball, smash in volleyball, kick in football, clearing the bar in the high jump and pole-vault, and hurdling, is built on the principles outlined above.

Notice that by keeping the left arm and both legs straight at the moment of shooting, the right hand will be raised to a maximal height (Figure 6.62).

In Figure 6.63 by holding both arms and right leg as high as possible, the left leg will reach the

Fig. 6.60

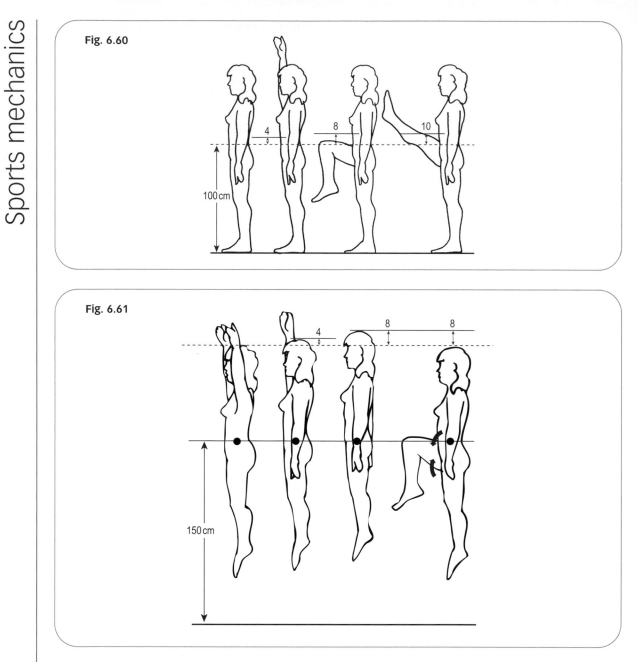

Fig. 6.61

ground at the earliest possible moment, and the hurdler can begin to run again.

Figure 6.64 further illustrates variations in CG location. Hip flexion causes the CG to vary in three different ways depending on the situation.

Figure 6.65A shows where the CG lies in a certain part of the body expressed as a percentage of its length. For example, the CG of the arm lies at a point which, measured from the shoulder downwards, corresponds to 40% of its length. The numbers shown in Figure 6.65B give the mass of each body part expressed as a percentage of total body weight. For example, the weight of the head is 7% that of the whole body weight.

The diagrams and calculations for Figure 6.66 show how we can make a total assessment of different exercises, once we know the location of the CG of a body, the body's moment of force and the function and position of its muscles.

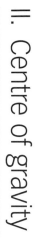

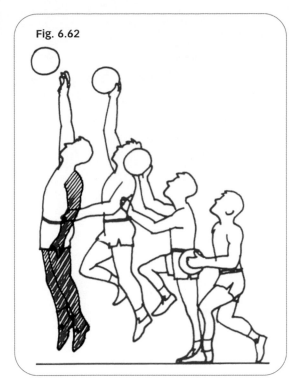

Fig. 6.62

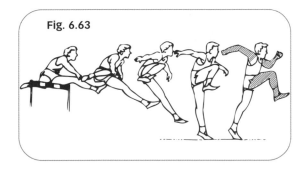

Fig. 6.63

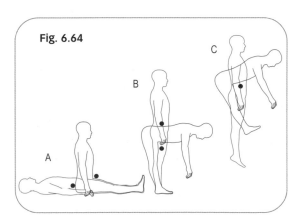

Fig. 6.64

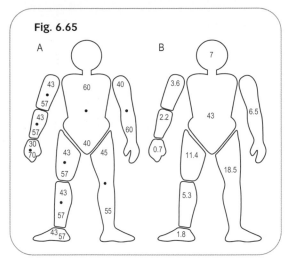

Fig. 6.65

Suppose a person hangs (Figure 6.66) so that the CG of her legs (45% of the leg's length from the hip) lies 0.40 m directly out from her hip in (A), 0.30 m in (B) and 0.30 m in (C). If her legs together weigh 25 kg (18.5% of her total body weight per leg), then the gravitational force acting on them will be 250 N.

Suppose the iliopsoas is the muscle holding the legs (Figure 6.67), and that its lever arm is 0.05 m.

Therefore, for the three positions in Figure 6.66:

(A)	(B)	(C)
$M = F \times l$	$M = F \times l$	$M = F \times l$
$M = 250 \times 0.40$	$M = 250 \times 0.30$	$M = 250 \times 0.30$
$M = 100$ Nm.	$M = 75$ Nm.	$M = 75$ Nm.

(A)	(B)	(C)
$F \times 0.05 = 100$	$F \times 0.05 = 75$	$F \times 0.05 = 75$
$F = 2000$ N.	$F = 1500$ N.	$F = 1500$ N.

All those who have tried position (B) in Figure 6.66 know that it is almost impossible to maintain, despite the fact that the muscle forces in (B)

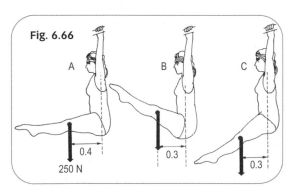

Fig. 6.66

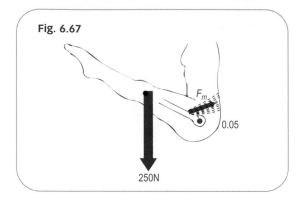

Fig. 6.67

F_m

0.05

250N

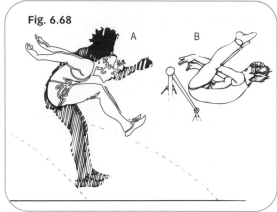

Fig. 6.68

A   B

and (C) are the same according to the calculations. However, the iliopsoas is longer in (C) than in (B), and thus more capable of exerting sufficient force. In (B) the distance between the origin and insertion of the muscle is perhaps less than 50% of its resting length. This means that the muscle cannot develop any force at all (p. 17). Another reason why it is 'impossible' to hold the legs in position (B), is that the hamstrings (p. 69) are so drawn out that they try to pull the legs down with great force much like an elastic band strives to return to its resting length.

In the situation shown in Figure 6.68, the interplay between hip flexion strength and hamstring flexibility is of decisive importance for the pattern of movement.

If the legs or upper body are folded forwards too early (Figure 6.68A), the legs cannot be held in the best position for landing. Instead, the body 'opens' so that the feet land too soon.

The following observation is made to illustrate further the CG concept and its importance. When a person lifts an object, different muscles will be engaged depending on how he moves the object.

If the lifts as in Figure 6.69A, the load to which his elbow flexors are subjected, will be less than if he lifts as shown in B (shorter lever arm (*l*)). The load to which the shoulder joint is subjected is almost zero in (A) but very large in (B).

Training the elbow flexors for strength, using a support for the upper arm (Figure 6.70), forces the elbow flexors to work the 'heavy way' and, at the same time, disengages the shoulder muscles.

It is easier to swing the legs forward more quickly if you first swing the legs back in the

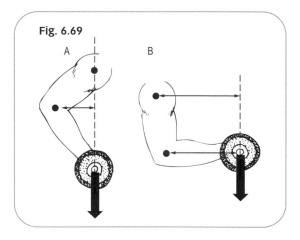

Fig. 6.69

A   B

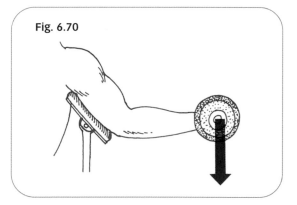

Fig. 6.70

opposite direction. From points 2 to 3 in Figure 6.71, the hip joints are extended in order to facilitate the the eccentric work of iliopsoas, which starts from a lengthened and strong position. Without this counter movement it is impossible to lift the legs and reach the position shown in 4 (indicated by a red dotted line), which is necessary to bring about this movement.

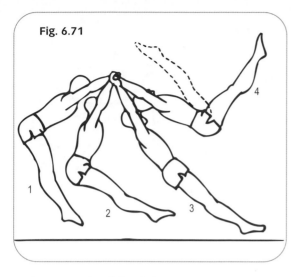

Fig. 6.71

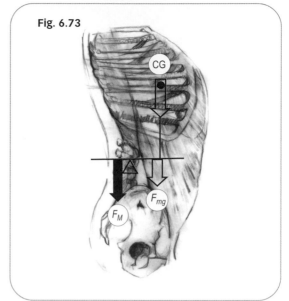

Fig. 6.73

Because the CG of the head lies a few centimetres in front of the upper cervical vertebra (Figure 6.72), the neck muscles are forced (F_M) to pull statically to hold the head. The CG of the upper body lies in front of the spine (Figure 6.73). Therefore, the back muscles are activated. The full weight of the trunk is concentrated on a point that lies a little in front of the hip joint (this varies greatly between individuals). Because of this, the buttock muscles are engaged (Figure 6.74). The quadriceps femoris (four-headed thigh muscle) counteracts the tendency of the body's weight to produce flexion at the knee joint. The soleus (flounder muscle), with the help of the gastrocnemius (twin calf muscle) counteracts the body's tendency to fall

forwards at the ankle joint (Figure 6.75). The function of all these muscles is to maintain the body's upright position. They are called postural muscles (Figures 6.72–6.75).

When a particular part of the body is to be moved, it is very important to be aware of the location of the CG. When an object is to be swung or whirled around, it can be shown that it is easier to initiate the movement when the radius of rotation is small. A hammer whose wire has a length of 0.5 m is easier to swing than one whose wire is, say, 1 m long. A hammer

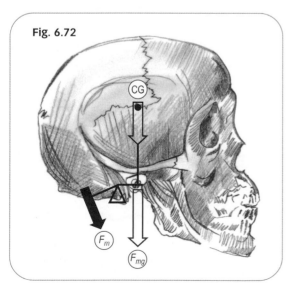

Fig. 6.72

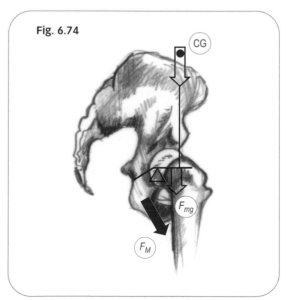

Fig. 6.74

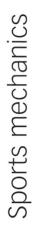
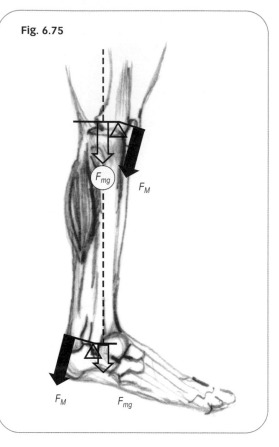

Fig. 6.75

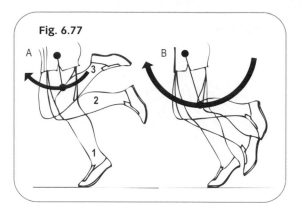

Fig. 6.77

hamstrings). Instead, they have time to allow the leg to swing forwards aided by the force of gravity and the hip flexors.

The arm is bent in the initial stage of almost any throwing or hitting event (Figure 6.78). As long as the shoulder muscles are accelerating the arm, the CG of the arm should be close to the shoulder. When throwing an object, muscle groups are activated in the order: abdomen, shoulder, elbow, wrist.

The pattern is the same when kicking a football (Figure 6.79). The muscles are then activated in the order: abdomen, hip, knee and foot.

On p. 141 it was pointed out that when two parts of a body of equal weight are brought together, they move symmetrically. This is only true when the distance between the CG and the joint is the same for both.

with a 3-m long wire-sling would be completely unmanageable (Figure 6.76).

If a person wants to swing his leg quickly forwards while running, it is important that he keep the swing radius as small as possible (Figure 6.77). This can be accomplished by pulling the heel up towards the buttock (3) as soon as the foot leaves the ground (1). The leg is then swung forwards with its CG as close as possible to the hip.

This type of running is typical for sprinters. Long-distance runners, on the other hand, do not waste energy by lifting the heel so high (which requires strength and speed of the

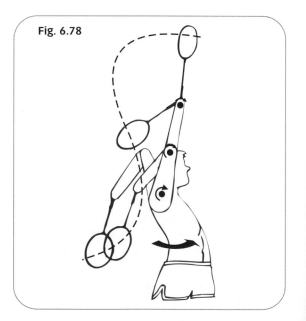

Fig. 6.78

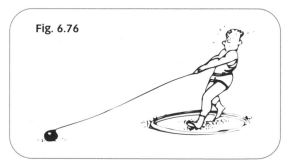

Fig. 6.76

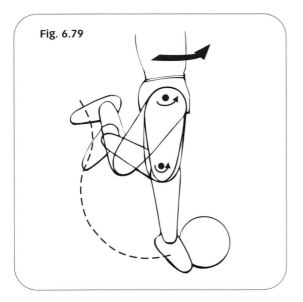

Fig. 6.79

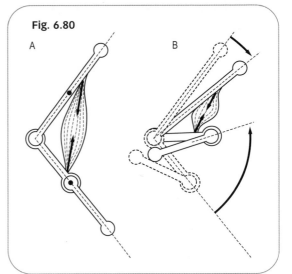

Fig. 6.80

If this is not the case, the part whose CG is farthest away from the joint will move through a smaller angle (Figure 6.80). This phenomenon is often used in athletics.

Thus, for effective movement at a joint, the parts of the joint should be arranged in such a way that the CG of the part to be moved lies close to the joint, while the CG of the others lie remote from it.

The following four examples (Figure 6.81A–D), in which the legs are swiftly swung forwards, illustrate this principle.

Example A. By maximally flexing the knee, the CG of the leg is brought to a point near the hip joint. This makes the leg easy to swing forwards. The CG of the upper body should, in principle, lie far from the hip joint, which implies that the arms should be relatively well flexed.

Example B. Before swinging his legs forward a long jumper first bends them maximally behind him (CG near the hips) and, at the same time, stretches his arms high above his head (CG far above the hips).

Example C. If a hurdler wants to make the most of the muscle force of his hip flexors, he should hold both his arms as far from his hips as possible (right arm straight, left arm bent for right leg to lead). His right leg should remain bent when his body is in the

rising phase of the jump and he should wait as long as possible before straightening it.

Example D. When a footballer heads the ball, his whole upper body should be moving quickly. Here, the CG of his upper body should lie near his hips (arms by his sides). The moment the ball is hit, the CG of his legs should lie far from his hips (straight

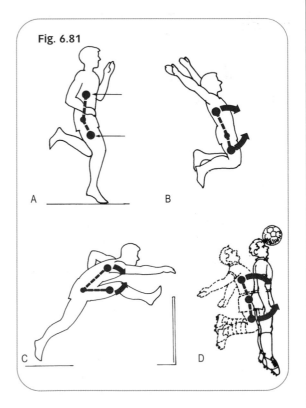

Fig. 6.81

A

B

C

D

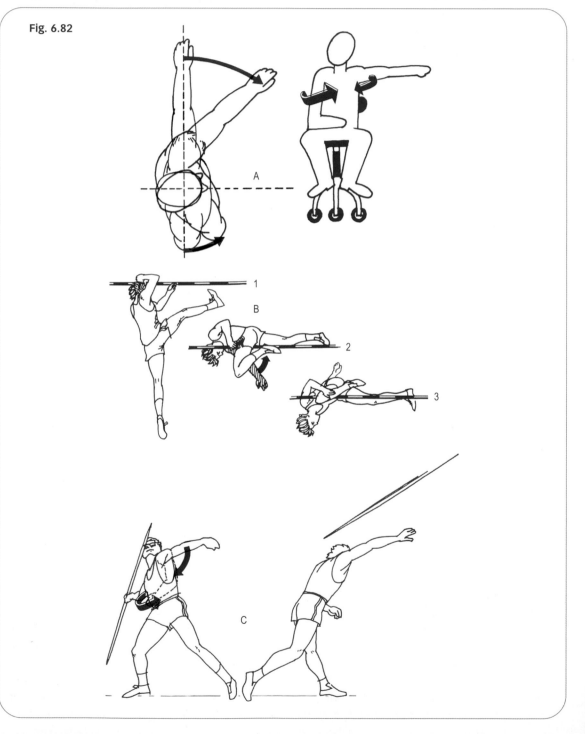

legs). Imagine how ineffective a header would be if made from a position corresponding to that shown in example B.

The following five examples (Figures 6.82 and 6.83) show how to arrange the body when making arm movements.

Figure 6.82:

Example A. If a person moves his arm in an arc in front of his body, his body will respond by rotating in the opposite direction. If his arm is bent, his body moves less. This and other similar effects can readily be observed

Fig. 6.82

with the aid of a mobile platform (turntable) or swivel chair.

Example B. To roll his trailing leg (left) over the bar in the straddle style high jump, the high jumper should pull his right arm in the opposite direction. Notice how the right arm changes position and rotates up behind the back in (2) and (3). The arm should be held straight and a long way from the body.

Example C. A straight arm that counters the rotation of the body is more effective for throwing than a bent arm that merely pulls in towards the body.

Figure 6.83A and B:

Example A. When landing the action of pulling the arms backwards and downwards causes the body to rotate in the opposite direction (or, the arm movements reduce the body rotation). As a result, the feet land further to the left than would be the case without arm movements.

Example B. If the arms are pulled down in front of the body, the feet will land further

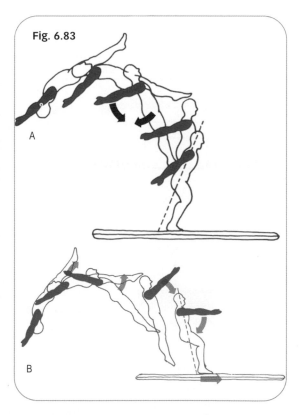

Fig. 6.83

A

B

to the right. This is due to the opposing arm movement. The muscles that pull the arms down arise from the chest and therefore must draw the body up. If the arms are kept straight, the opposing movement of the body is greater than if the arms are bent. If the arms are pulled outwards and downwards no counter movements will be produced.

III. Acceleration

Newton's second law, which was mentioned on p. 133, states that every force that acts on an object tries to accelerate the object.

Definition:

Acceleration is change of velocity per time period.

This can be written in a formula:

$$a = (v_1 - v_0)/(t_1 - t_0)$$

t_0 is the time when you start to observe the movement.

t_1 is the time when you finish observing the movement.

v_0 is the initial velocity.

v_1 is the final velocity.

Acceleration is measured, according to the definition, in metre/second/second, expressed as m/s^2. Examples of how to use the formula of acceleration:

1. A 100 metres runner reaches a velocity of 10 m/s after 4.0 s. How great is the acceleration during this time?
   The formula gives: $a = (10 - 0)/(4.0 - 0)$; $a = 10/4$; $a = 2.5$. Result: 2.5 m/s^2.
2. The same runner had reached the velocity of 4.0 m/s already after 1.0 s. How large was a during this first second?
   The formula gives $a = (4.0 - 0)/(1.0 - 0)$; $a = 4.0$ m/s^2. Result: 4.0 m/s^2.

The acceleration is greater during the first step than later on in the race because the muscles in the legs can develop more force directed towards the ground at this stage, when the time span for the muscle contraction is long (the runner runs at a slower pace) as opposed to when the time span for the contraction is short (the runner runs at a faster pace). You will find the principal correlation between force and contraction velocity in a muscle on p. 21.

During the first step the force available is just to the right of the isometric maximum. The faster the speed is the lower the forces will be and therefore acceleration will be lower. The greatest acceleration takes place during the very first step (Figure 6.84).

If we suppose that a sprinter shoots away at the first step with a force of 2000 N, in the direction shown in Figure 6.84A, only that part of the force directed forward (F_h) will give acceleration. F_v will raise the sprinter's centre of gravity. In step number two the total force will be a little smaller as seen in Figure 6.84B. This together with the fact that the direction of the thrust is somewhat more upright means that F_h becomes smaller and that the acceleration forwards will be lower in the second step than in the first step.

During free fall, when you disregard air resistance the acceleration of the body is always 9.81 m/s². Newton stated this in the late seventeenth century after having conducted a series of experiments involving weights, following on from Galileo's earlier work. He dropped 1 kg from different heights, measured the time for the fall and found that the acceleration during the fall was always 9.81 m/s². When he dropped 5 kg or 10 kg weights the result was still the same:

$a = 9.81$ m/s².

He then hypothesized that, on every kilogram, the earth acts with an attractive force of 9.81 N, a force unit that can be used to summarize all his experiments in one single formula, namely Newton's second law.

$$F = m \times a$$

where m (mass) is measured in kilograms, a (acceleration) in m/s² and F (force) in newtons (N).

Notes from Newton's tests could have looked like those in Figure 6.85.

Test 1: The mass 1.0 kg falls freely. The velocity after 1.0 s was measured at exactly 9.81 m/s.

According to the formula $a = (v_1 - v_0)/(t_1 - t_0)$, he could first calculate a to be 9.81 m/s² and then with the help of $F = m \times a$, he could say that F must have been 9.81 N.

Make the calculations for the other three tests as well.

Figure 6.86 will be used to explain what happens when an object that is lying on a flat surface is moved away by a pulling force. Suppose that F is 300 N. What happens?

The object weighs 10 kg and is pulled towards the ground with a gravitational force of 100 N. The ground repels the object with a force, that is called the normal force, which is also 100 N.

Fig. 6.85

mass	time	velocity	acc.	force
1	1	9.81	9.81	9.81
2	2	19.92	9.81	19.62
10	3	30	10	100
6	0.5	5	10	60

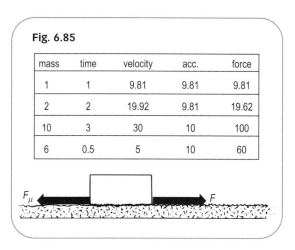

Fig. 6.84

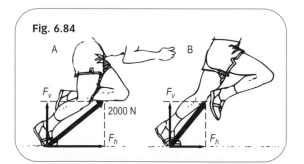

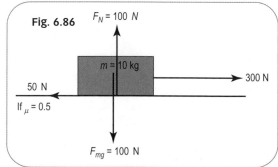

F_μ is the force of friction directed to the left, which, on this occasion, tries to prevent a movement to the right. If the normal force (F_N) is 100 N and $\mu = 0.5$, fully developed friction is 50 N. The formula used is:

$$F_\mu = \mu \times F_N.$$

In this section we will discuss how the force of friction applies to an object's acceleration (if you wish to refamiliarize yourself with the concept of friction, see p. 142). In the example above, the pulling force is 300 N and the force of friction is 50 N. The accelerating force will therefore be $300 - 50 = 250$ N.

The formula $F = m \times a$ gives $250 = 10 \times a$; $a = 25$ m/s^2.

If the box is pulled for 0.2 s the box would reach a velocity of $v = a \times t$. In other words $v = 25 \times 0.2$; $v = 5.0$ m/s.

Exercise 1. Calculate the acceleration and the final velocity if all values are the same as in Figure 6.86 except for the pulling force which is changed to 120 N.

Result: $a = 7$ m/s^2; $v = 1.4$ m/s.

Exercise 2. Suppose that 5.0 kg is added to the top of the box. You now pull with 300 N, as in the original example. What will the values a and v become?

Result: $a = 15$ m/s^2; $v = 3.0$ m/s.

Exercise 3. Suppose that the box weighs 60 kg, the force of friction is 0.2 and the pulling force is 150 N. Calculate a and v.

Result: $a = 0.5$ m/s^2; $v = 0.1$ m/s.

Exercise 4. Suppose that the box weighs 100 kg, the friction coefficient is 0.4 and the pulling force is 800 N. Calculate a and v.

Result: $a = 4.0$ m/s^2; $v = 0.8$ m/s.

Exercise 5. Suppose that the box weighs 40 kg, the friction coefficient is 0.1 and the pulling force is 30 N. What happens?

Result: The box stands still. (You have to exceed 40 N before the box starts moving.)

IV. Impulse and momentum

If the force equation ($F = m \times a$) is rewritten according to the following: $F = m \times a$ multiplied by t gives:

$F \times t = m \times a \times t$ and since $a \times t = v$:

$F \times t = m \times v$

This use of the force equation takes into consideration the time over which a force is acting. The velocity (v) that is achieved during this time can be directly determined. As often happens within the field of physics, the behaviour and properties of bodies are described by several independent concepts.

Impulse

The left side in the formula above, $F \times t$, is called impulse.

$F \times t = $ Impulse

If a body is acted on by a force (F) during a certain time (t), the body has received an impulse. The magnitude of the impulse depends on the size of F and t and it is measured in units called Newton-seconds (Ns).

Example 1. If a sprinter pushes off with a force of 2000 N over 0.1 s the impulse is $2000 \times 0.1 = 200$ Ns.
Example 2. A gravitational force of 600 N is acting on a diver over 1.2 s. The impulse obtained is 720 Ns.

Momentum

The right side in the equation $F \times t = m \times v$ is called momentum.

$m \times v = $ momentum

Example 3. A basketball that weighs 0.5 kg and moves with a velocity of 15 m/s has a momentum of $mv = 0.5 \times 15 = 7.5$ kg m/s.
Example 4. If the sprinter in Example 1 weighs 50 kg the push-away step will give him a velocity of $2000 \times 0.1 = 50 \times v$; $200 = 50 \times v$; $v = 4$ m/s. The momentum is 200 kg m/s.

Example 5. A high jumper who swings an arm straight up at the jump has given the arm a momentum of 15 kg m/s if the arm weighs 5 kg and the arm's centre of gravity has a velocity of 3 m/s at the moment of take-off.

$$F \times t = m \times v$$

The formula $Ft = mv$ states that an impulse gives a momentum.

The formula can also be read the other way around: a momentum can be transformed into an impulse.

Example 6. To completely brake a body that has a momentum of 1500 kg m/s takes an impulse of 1500 Ns.

Example 7. A gymnast weighing 60 kg lands from a jump with a velocity of 5 m/s (Figure 6.87). The braking time is supposed to be 0.2 s. When he stands still he has lost all his momentum. We can then calculate the mean value of the force that caused the stop. We assume that the jumper is standing still after the landing.

$$m \times v = F \times t$$

$m \times v = F \times t$ gives $60 \times 5 = F \times 0.2$
$300 = F \times 0.2$, $F = 1500N$

The average braking force was 1500 N.

The concept of impulse is used to describe how a body is influenced by a force. There are many situations in sports where forces acting over short or long periods affect either the sportsman or the sports equipment. For example, the initial thrust of a sprinter, the take-off in the long jump, a racket hitting a ball and the thrust developed in swimming strokes.

The concept of momentum also comes into use in describing how body parts and equipment move. A heavy ball with a low speed can be more difficult to catch than a light ball travelling faster. To be tackled by a light person moving at high speed during an ice-hockey game might not be as bad as being tackled by a heavy player moving more slowly. It is the degree of momentum that is crucial. The following can be used as a template on which to base discussions of these situations.

A medicine ball that weighs 4.0 kg comes towards me at 5 m/s. The momentum of the ball is $mv = 20$ kg m/s. The impulse required to stop the ball must therefore be 20 Ns. Assume the braking time to be 0.05 s, $20 = F \times 0.05$, $F = 20/0.05$, $F = 400$ N.

Braking the medicine ball forces the triceps brachii muscles to work eccentrically with an average force of 400 N (see Figure 6.88, plot (a)).

If I receive the ball in a more yielding fashion, so that the braking time is doubled, then the braking force will be halved, that is it will be 200 N (Figure 6.88 plot (b)). The impulse is often described by drawing a diagram that shows how the force (F) and the time (t) depend on each other. The two variants of receiving the medicine ball can then be described by the graphs in Figure 6.88.

The magnitude of the impulse that acts on the body corresponds to size of the area below the lines (a) and (b) in Figure 6.88. The larger the area the larger the impulse.

In reality, the force that is used to receive the ball is not a constant 400 N during the braking

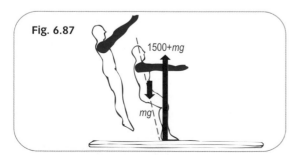

Fig. 6.87

1500+*mg*

mg

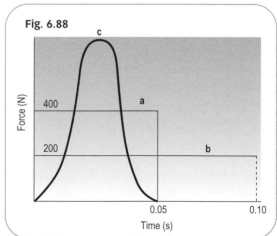

Fig. 6.88

Force (N)

400

200

0.05   0.10

Time (s)

process; it grows from zero up to a maximum and then decreases. 400 N is the average braking force. A more realistic braking curve would therefore look like that in Figure 6.88(c).

Notice, however, that the areas under all three curves are the same.

The curves in Figure 6.89 show two different impulse diagrams experienced by a person weighing 45 kg. In each case, the normal force is shown when he is running and walking. In each case, the area under the curve is equal to the impulse experienced by the person during contact with the ground.

The concept of momentum is often used to explain what happens when a body collides with or adheres to another body. In Figure 6.90 a moving wagon comes along with a mass m_1 and a velocity u_1. The wagon collides with another wagon with a mass m_2 that has a velocity u_2. When the wagons collide there will be a force on one of the wagons in one direction and an equal collinear force acting on the other wagon (obeying Newton's law of action–reaction forces). One of the wagons receives an impulse from the other, that is one of the wagons increases its momentum by exactly as much as the other loses momentum.

At the time of impact, the momentum is conserved.

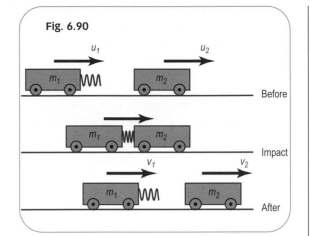

Fig. 6.90

Using symbols for mass and velocity this can be written:

$$m_1u_1 + m_2u_2 = m_1v_1 + m_2v_2$$

Momentum of force before impact = momentum after impact.
(u = the original velocity and v = the final velocity.) The formula applies for all values of masses and velocities.

Figures 6.90 and 6.91 show situations in which the momentum is conserved. In Figure 6.91, if the man pushes the boy so that he moves backwards with velocity 0.40 m/s, the following applies.

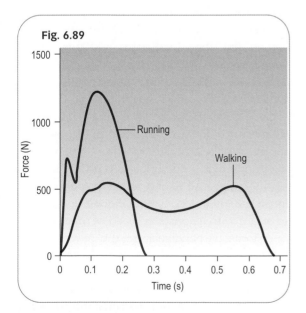

Fig. 6.89

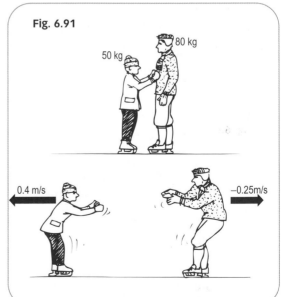

Fig. 6.91

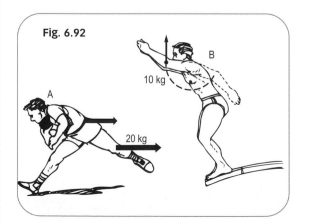

$$(50 \times 0) + (80 \times 0) = (50 \times 0.4) + (80 \times v_l)$$
$$0 = 20 + (80 \times v_l)$$
$$v_l = -20/80, \, v_l = -0.25 \text{ m/s}$$

The man moves away with a velocity of 0.25 m/s in the opposite direction to the boy.

Suppose that the athlete in Figure 6.92A thrusts his left leg, which weighs 20 kg, straight backwards at a velocity of 5.0 m/s. When the leg is completely outstretched it will 'drag' the rest of the body, which weighs 80 kg. The leg will be halted and will lose momentum. The body will, however, take over exactly as much momentum as the leg will lose. The calculation is as follows:

$$(20 \times 5.0) + (80 \times 0) = 100 \times v_l$$
$$100 = 100 \times v_l$$
$$v_l = 1.0 \text{ m/s}$$

The whole body will move at a velocity of 1.0 m/s straight backwards in the pushing direction.

The athlete has imparted velocity to his body, and thereby to the shot, via his left leg, even though it does not have contact with the ground. The contribution from the left leg adds to the force generated by the velocity of the right leg, the rotation of the body and the extension of the arm.

In Figure 6.92B it can be seen how the arms contribute to the height of the jump by adding their momentum to the whole body at take-off.

The expression for conservation of momentum can also explain the phenomenon that is indicated in Figure 6.93. If you stand up and walk straight forwards in a boat that is not

Fig. 6.93

moving, the boat will glide backwards. Before the man starts to walk to the right the momentum is zero. The man moves forwards with help from friction against the boards of the boat. During every step the boat is acted on with an impulse ($F \times t$) whose magnitude is directly proportional to the size of the man. In other words, the boat gains a backward momentum which is equal to the forward momentum gained by the person. The total momentum is still zero. If the boat is a great deal heavier than the person it will glide away slowly from the jetty; if it is much lighter it will glide away faster than the person can walk, and then…(what will happen?)

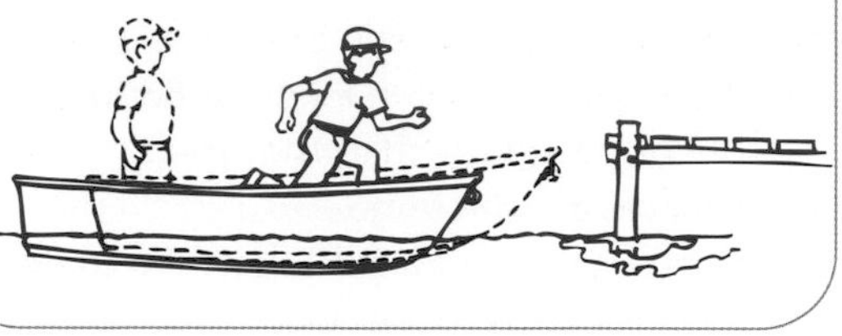

V. Circular motion

Until now we have mainly looked at bodies moving straight ahead (linear movement). The expressions and the examples we have used have not described what makes bodies turn away from a linear path. There is a difference between movements where something is rotating on the spot (pirouette) and movements where something follows a circular path. The latter is usually called circular motion; with this type of motion you usually describe how fast the rotation is by indicating, for example, number of rotations per minute, number of degrees per second or as appropriate for the situation.

A body that is not influenced by any force at all, i.e. where all acting forces are equal, will move linearly at a constant velocity, or continue to rotate with a constant speed of rotation.

A force perpendicular to the movement of the body will compel the body to move in a circle.

To ensure that a circular trajectory is described, the force must be constantly directed

Fig. 6.92

towards the centre of the circle. The magnitude of the force (F_c) determines the radius (r) for a body with a certain mass (m) and a certain velocity (v). The force is called <u>centripetal</u> force F_c. The correlation between the different physical quantities is:

$$F_c = m \times v^2/r$$

Example 1. To swing a hammer that weighs 7 kg (Figure 6.94) in a circular course of radius 2 m and with a velocity of 20 m/s, the inwardly directed force F_c has to be:

$$F_c = m \times v^2/r = 7 \times 20^2/2 = 1400 \text{ N}.$$

Example 2. When a downhill-skier negotiates a sharp turn (Figure 6.95) he is, for a moment, describing a circular course. If the skier weighs 70 kg, the radius of the turn he makes is 15 m, and he has a velocity of 10 m/s, the inward directed force is:

$$F_c = 70 \times 10^2/15 = 467 \text{ N}$$

In both these examples it takes a great deal of strength to manage the loads that are placed on the legs. In skiing the load is mainly on the outer leg in the turn. This leg is a lot straighter at the knee joint and is therefore able to thrust more than the inner leg, which is more bent and thereby in a very poor position to give any support to the centripetal force.

When running straight ahead, to turn off in another direction (Figure 6.96) you must place the outer foot to the side of the earlier running direction in order to initiate the turn. It is the inward-directed component of the force of friction that functions as the centripetal force. In the figure it can be seen how the feet steer in the wrong direction to generate a force directed inwards.

When analysing a sharp turn in downhill-skiing, ice-skating or cycling one can also see that sometimes the tracks show an initiating turn made apparently in the 'wrong direction'. This, however, causes the body to lean inwards to achieve the position that is needed to maintain balance and create the right centripetal force.

As seen in the figures above, different types of force can act centripetally. In Figure 6.94, it is the pulling force from the thrower. In Figure 6.95, it is the force of friction against the snow. In Figures 6.99 and Figure 6.100 it is the normal force and the force from the fingers that act as the centripetal force.

When analysing sports movements that involve curved trajectories, the concept of centrifugal force is often used – but it is often used wrongly. It must to be made clear that:

Centrifugal force does not exist.

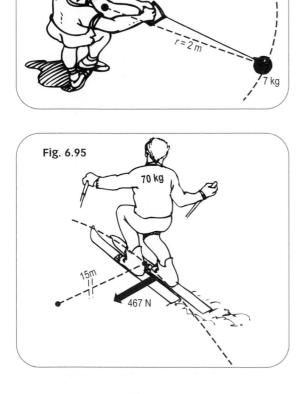

Fig. 6.94

$r = 2$ m

7 kg

Fig. 6.95

70 kg

15 m

467 N

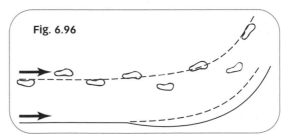

Fig. 6.96

Centrifugal force is a fictitious force invented by physicists to make certain calculations easier. To explain this we will look at two different situations that are familiar.

Suppose that you hang a 'mascot' in the ceiling of a car. When the car is travelling straight ahead at a constant speed (or is immobile), the mascot will hang straight down. When the car accelerates forward something happens (Figure 6.97).

The fastening point of the mascot's suspension thread starts to move faster but the mascot moves at the same speed as before. Almost immediately after the acceleration has begun, the thread will pull on the mascot and vice-versa so that the thread is swinging 'forwards' in the air. The pulling force in the thread has become larger and the forward component has a magnitude sufficiently large to accelerate the mascot to the same extent as the car.

If you sit inside the car and accelerate together with the car it is convenient to say that the mascot is swinging backwards, but in fact it is not. The mascot only moves forwards. During a brief interval before the thread has become stretched the car travels away from the mascot. If you imagine that the car is standing still you can invent a fictitious force and say that the mascot is acted on by a backward force. However, this is not reality.

The real force is directed forward. If you look at what happens when a vehicle with a mascot hanging from the ceiling turns in a curve after having driven straight ahead (Figure 6.98) you can see the following: the mascot is hanging straight down when the vehicle is driving straight ahead at a constant speed. When the driver turns the steering wheel there will be a force of friction on

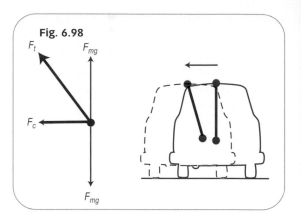

Fig. 6.98

the tyres that will be directed towards the centre of the curve. The fastening point for the mascot follows at the very beginning of the turn, but not the mascot, since it is not acted on by any force. Immediately after the turning begins the thread pulls the mascot along. Seen from the outside the mascot has not been acted on outwardly in the turn; instead it has just continued to move straight forwards until the tension in the thread pulls it into the same turn as the vehicle. The force in the thread can be divided into two different components, one of them equal to the weight of the mascot and the other to the centripetal force, which, according to the above formula makes the mascot describe the same turn as the vehicle.

Without the force of friction the vehicle cannot turn. Without the inward-directed pulling force in the thread the mascot will not be pulled along by the thread.

There are actually no outwardly directed forces acting on either the vehicle or the mascot. Nevertheless, there will seem to be if you sit inside the turning car. You can then describe the events as if the mascot is swinging outward in the turn. This can be explained by a fictitious force called centrifugal force.

Fictitious forces, which are described above, are used only to explain actions within accelerating systems. In connection with sports it is, most of the time, irrelevant to use fictitious terms. As far as I know, there are no sports activities taking place inside cars, buses, elevators or spaceships that accelerate at the same time as the athlete is performing his activities. To change the movement of a body it takes a force in a desired

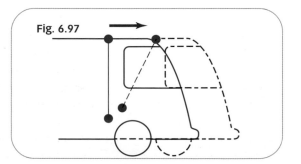

Fig. 6.97

direction and nothing else. Collinear forces acting on the body don't exist. Here, follow some more examples that describe the force situation when different bodies are changing direction.

Example 1. In a slanting curve the centripetal force derives from the normal force, which has an inward-directed component. Trotting-tracks, indoor-tracks with sharp turns, and cycle velodromes (Figure 6.99) are all built with an incline so that the inwardly directed component of the normal force will be just right to get the object in the desired course. F_v will be just right to counterbalance mg.

Example 2. If a gymnast (weight 70 kg) hangs still on a horizontal bar (Figure 6.100),

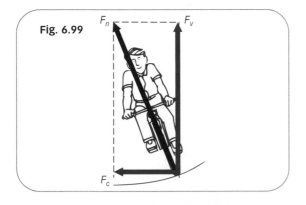

Fig. 6.99

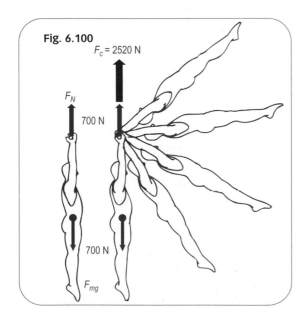

Fig. 6.100

he is acted on by the force of gravity F_{mg} and normal force F_N

These forces are equal (700 N) and collinear. If he, on the other hand, is going to do a so-called giant swing at a speed of 6.0 m/s and with his CG following a circular path with a radius of 1.0 m, the required centripetal force is 2520 N. That is:

$$F_c = m \times v^2/r; \; F_c = 70 \times 6^2/1 = 70 \times 36 = 2520 \text{ N}.$$

The total force is then:

$$2520 + 700 = 3220 \text{ N}.$$

VI. Moment of inertia

The previous examples show that the further from the centre of rotation that the centre of gravity of a particular part of the body lies, the greater is the force required of the muscles to set the body part in motion. Of course, the mass (weight) of the body part is also important. The more the body part weighs, the more force is required to set it in motion (or stop it from moving).

In physics, the term moment of inertia is used to describe the combination of the weight of a body and how far from the axis of rotation its centre of gravity lies. The figures in the left-hand column of Figure 6.101 have lower moments of inertia than their counterparts in the right-hand column.

In physics the letter I is used to symbolize moment of inertia. In order to determine the moment of inertia of a body we must know its mass (m) and its rotational radius (r). The moment of inertia is:

$$I = mr^2$$

The underlined numbers in Figure 6.102 give an idea of how much force must be exerted in order to set the different bodies in motion.

If we want to calculate the moment of inertia of a body rotating about its own centre of gravity (which happens in all flights through the air), we make the calculation shown in Figure 6.103.

It has been shown with this type of calculation that the moment of inertia for rotation about a

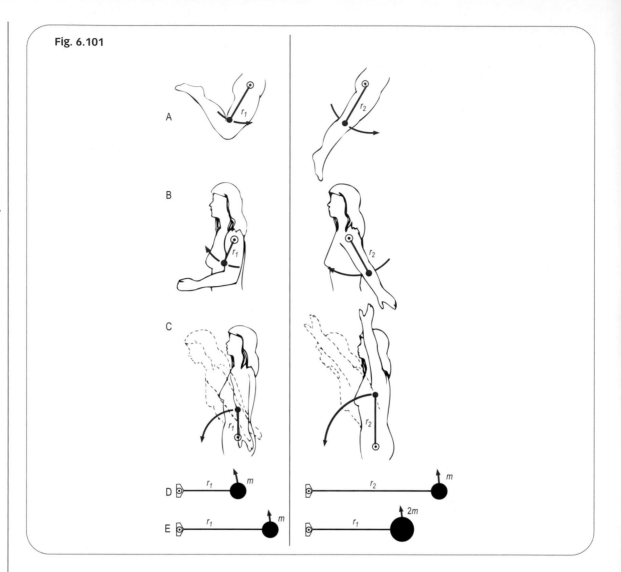

Fig. 6.101

body's longitudinal axis varies as the body takes up different positions. In Figure 6.104 variations in body position are compared with the anatomical position (I). Realistic values for that position in 6.103 are in the range 1.0–1.2 kgm^2.

The moment of inertia will increase as more body segments move away from the longitudinal axis of rotation, i.e. as the distance (r) to the axis increases.

The moment of inertia for forward and backward rotation (vault) varies roughly according to the data presented in Figure 6.105.

It has been shown by experiment that when a body is made to rotate by some force and thereafter left to rotate without being influenced by other external forces, its rotational velocity (ω) will depend on its body position. It is said that moment of inertia × rotational velocity does not change. $I \times \omega =$ constant. This has the following consequences.

Example 1. If a person who is rotating with his arms by his sides (I) at a certain rotational velocity (ω) lifts his arms out, he will reduce his rotational velocity by half ($\omega/2$). The moment of inertia will be changed from I to $2I$ by this change in his position. The values I, $2I$ and $4I$ are taken from Figure 6.104. If he sinks down to a half-sitting position, I will be changed to $4I$, and hence his rotational velocity (ω) is reduced to a quarter ($\omega/4$). An example of another change is provided by the execution of a pirouette

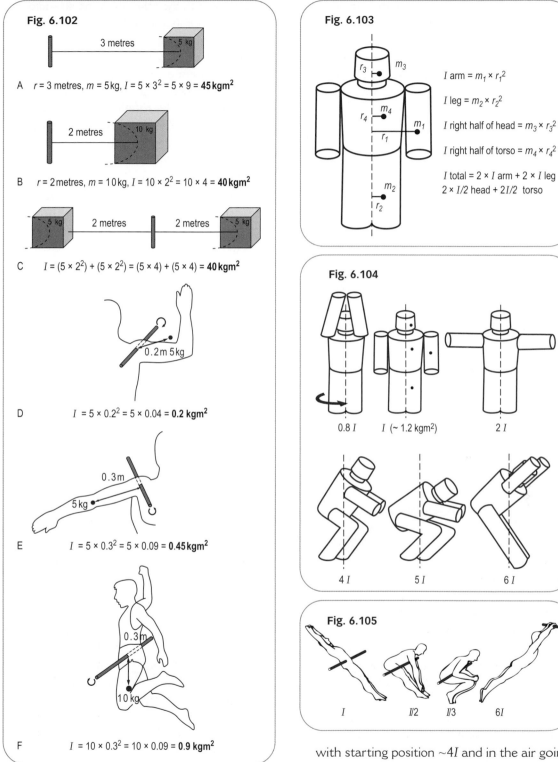

Fig. 6.102

A $r = 3$ metres, $m = 5$ kg, $I = 5 \times 3^2 = 5 \times 9 = \mathbf{45\,kgm^2}$

B $r = 2$ metres, $m = 10$ kg, $I = 10 \times 2^2 = 10 \times 4 = \mathbf{40\,kgm^2}$

C $I = (5 \times 2^2) + (5 \times 2^2) = (5 \times 4) + (5 \times 4) = \mathbf{40\,kgm^2}$

D $I = 5 \times 0.2^2 = 5 \times 0.04 = \mathbf{0.2\;kgm^2}$

E $I = 5 \times 0.3^2 = 5 \times 0.09 = \mathbf{0.45\,kgm^2}$

F $I = 10 \times 0.3^2 = 10 \times 0.09 = \mathbf{0.9\;kgm^2}$

Fig. 6.103

I arm $= m_1 \times r_1^2$

I leg $= m_2 \times r_2^2$

I right half of head $= m_3 \times r_3^2$

I right half of torso $= m_4 \times r_4^2$

I total $= 2 \times I$ arm $+ 2 \times I$ leg
$2 \times I/2$ head $+ 2I/2$ torso

Fig. 6.104

0.8 I I (~ 1.2 kgm²)   2 I

4 I 5 I 6 I

Fig. 6.105

I $I/2$ $I/3$ 6I

with starting position ~4I and in the air going down to ~2I or as low as ~I (Figure 6.106). *Example 2.* In certain kinds of turns in skiing, the skier starts from a deep position (e.g. 4I) and stands during the swing (2I). He thus

171

roughly doubles his initial rotation (Figure 6.107).

When coming out of a turn, the skier can reduce his rotational velocity to about a half by dropping down to a deeper position from 2*I* to 4*I*. Hence, he will find it easier to steer straight again (Figure 6.108).

Example 3. In the take-off in the straddle style high-jump, the body reaches a position of great rotational inertia about an axis that is parallel to the bar (Figure 6.109A). If the jumper cannot quickly change his position, he risks knocking the bar off with his trailing leg. This is because his rotation is very slow in this position. When he comes to straddle the bar with his trailing leg, it is important that his rotational velocity is at a maximum, i.e. the moment of inertia should be minimal. He ensures this by keeping his body straight and his arms close to his sides (Figure 6.109B).

Example 4. The flop-style high jumper rotates backwards with greater speed if he arches his back than if his body is straight. At the same time he has better stability against sideways rotation if he holds his arms out than if he keeps them close to his body (Figure 6.110).

Example 5. A thrower increases the total rotational velocity of his body (and thus the

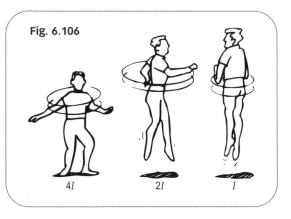

Fig. 6.106

4*I*   2*I*   *I*

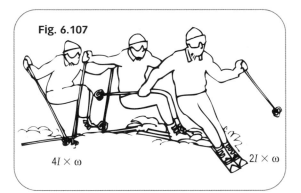

Fig. 6.107

4*I* × ω   2*I* × ω

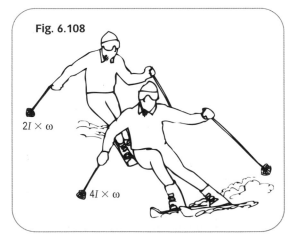

Fig. 6.108

2*I* × ω

4*I* × ω

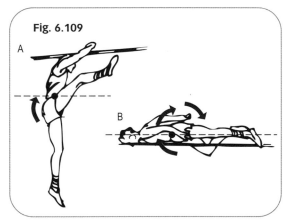

Fig. 6.109

A

B

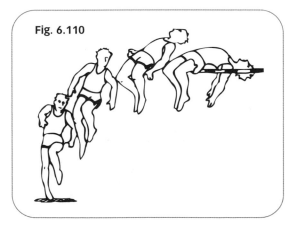

Fig. 6.110

velocity of his throwing arm) in the following way. In the final phase of the throw, he rises from a relatively low position to one that centres all the parts of his body – except his throwing arm – around the rotational axis (Figure 6.111).

Example 6. A swimmer starts a front crawl flip turn by flipping his legs down against the water (which resists by pressing up against him as shown by the arrows in Figure 6.112). His hands also press in the wrong direction. By piking at the hip, he makes the water press against his back. These three expedients give him a certain rotational velocity (ω). At this point, he folds his trunk maximally, thereby doubling the rotational velocity he has already acquired.

Example 7. A gymnast who wishes to rotate about a bar (wheel swing) has greater difficulty in swinging around it if her body is kept completely straight (Figure 6.113A) than if there is slight piking at the hips B. By piking slightly she shifts her centre of gravity (CG) to a location remote from her body, i.e. near the bar. If she tries to swing around the bar by pulling her head backwards, that is by arching slightly, her difficulties will only increase (C).

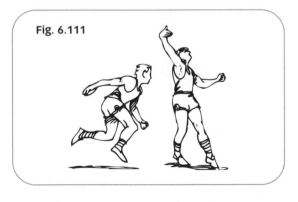

Fig. 6.111

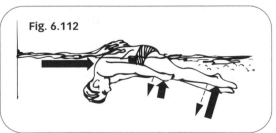

Fig. 6.112

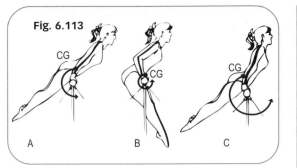

Fig. 6.113

In the discussion above, we assume that the girl has already created a certain speed of rotation (ω).

When a body rotates, its rotational velocity can be expressed by specifying for example how many revolutions per minute it completes or how many degrees per second it rotates.

Another unit for rotational velocity is radian/second. One radian/second means that something rotates such that the length a point (A) moves is one radius every second. A radian equals approximately 57.3°. (Since the circumference of a circle is $O = 2\pi$ it will take 2π radians, that is 2×3.14 radians = 6.28 radians, to complete a full circle. 6.28 radians = 360° 1 radian = 360°/6.28 = 57.3°.) (Figure 6.114).

Figure 6.115A–C shows three bodies that gain rotation from different forces. These three bodies could have been acted on by exactly the same torque but will behave differently, i.e turn at different speeds after the torque has finished. This depends on the bodies having different moments of inertia. The one that has the smallest moment of inertia (I) starts to rotate the fastest. The correlation between the torque ($M = F \times l$) and the

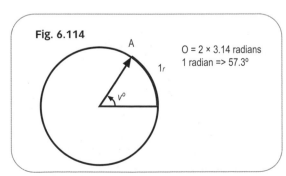

Fig. 6.114

$O = 2 \times 3.14$ radians
1 radian => 57.3°

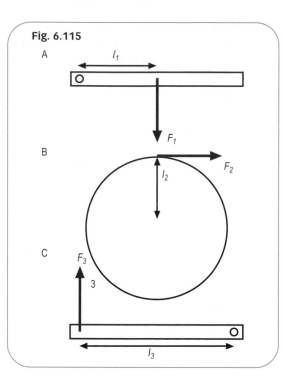

Fig. 6.115

you can grab something next to you to generate force from outside. The force by which you create the rotation (F), the distance from the platform centre that the force is acting (l) and the time over which the force is acting (t) give $F \times l \times t$ in the formula above. You have created angular momentum (H). How much rotational velocity is created depends on the magnitude of the moment of inertia of the platform and of the person standing on it ($I \times \omega$). When the forces have finished acting on you, you will have changed body position and therefore you will also have a different inertia (I), which means that your velocity of rotation (ω) will also have changed.

Suppose that Figure 6.117 shows what happens after you have commenced rotation with the help of an external force.

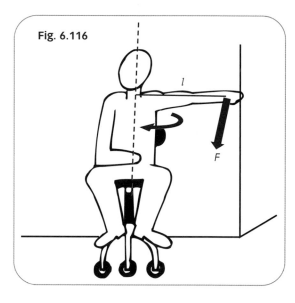

Fig. 6.116

moment of inertia (I) is analagous to that between force and mass in linear motion:

Linear movement	Angular movement
$F = m \times a$	$M = I \times \alpha$
(a is linear acceleration.)	(α is angular acceleration.)
If the force F acts for t seconds you can write	If the moment M acts for t seconds you can write
$F \times t = m \times a \times t$	$M \times t = I \times \alpha \times t$
or	or
$F \times t = m \times v$ (since $a \times t = v$)	$M \times t = I \times \omega$ (since $\alpha \times t = \omega$)
$F \times t$ is called momentum	$M \times t$ is called angular momentum, which is sometimes denoted by H ($H = I \times \omega$)

To show in practice what H is and how it works you can imagine a platform which, with the aid of ball bearings, rotates easily (a piano-chair would also serve).

To generate rotation an external force is required. Someone can help you to get going or

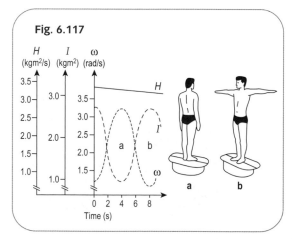

Fig. 6.117

H, from the left axis, is approximately 3.4 kgm²/s at the beginning and decreases slowly to 3.2 kgm²/s after 10 seconds. H decreases due to the friction from the platform's ball bearings and slight air resistance against the body's movement. Without these forces the angular momentum would remain constant at 3.4 kgm²/s for an infinite time. In practice there are always external forces that 'steal' from the angular momentum. In the other two graphs you can also see that when the arms are outstretched (b) the moment of inertia (I) is approximately 2.8 kgm²/s and the rotational velocity is approximately 1.2 m/s.

$$H = I \times \omega \qquad\qquad 3.4 = 2.8 \times 1.2$$

When the arms are hanging (a) along the side of the body, I is only 1.0 which gives a rotational velocity of approximately 3.4, everything obeying

$$H = I \times \omega \qquad\qquad 3.4 = 1.0 \times 3.4$$

The following analogy might help you to understand the formula

$$\boldsymbol{F \times l \times t = I \times \omega}$$

Suppose that you fill a U-tube with some water (Figure 6.118). One half of the tube represents I and the other side represents ω. Pouring the water imparts a rotation: force (F) works with a lever (l) during a certain period of time (t).

The greater $F \times l \times t$, the more water there is in the U-tube. You can now, with help from a piston, regulate the height of the water-pillars. The lower I is, the higher ω will be. The more water (H) from the beginning the greater rotational velocity (the higher the water-pillar in the right tube) with help from the piston.

In practice the U-tube leaks (compare with air resistance and friction that decrease H).

Imagine you are going to carry out a volleyball service action as depicted in Figure 6.119, and that, in so doing, you impart rotation to the arm.

The formula $F \times l \times t = I \times \omega$ will describe the following: F is the force whereby one or a few muscles pull your arm. l is the lever for the muscle around the centre of the shoulder joint. t is the time over which the muscle is acting on the arm. I is the arm's torque, and ω is the rotational velocity that has been built up during the action of the muscle. The deltoideus (deltoid muscle) has the main responsibility for the movement in a forearm-serve in volleyball.

Further examples of how to initiate rotation are given below.

When a dancer does a preparation jump for a pirouette (6.120) the rotational velocity will depend on the force of friction (F_μ) against the floor. The lever l is the distance from the force to the rotational centre, which is directly below CG.

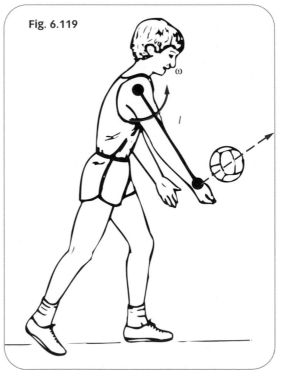

Fig. 6.119

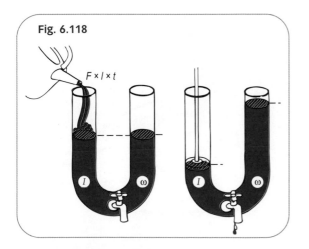

Fig. 6.118

$F \times l \times t$

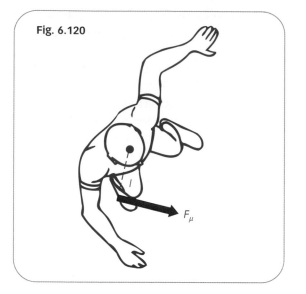

Fig. 6.120

F_μ

t is the time over which the force is acting before the dancer leaves the floor. If the arms are held far away from the body, the preparation will go more slowly, so *t* will be longer and the initial value of the angular momentum will be larger. If the arms are held remote from the body the dancer can pull them in and thereby increase the rotational velocity in the air compared to the velocity that was achieved when leaving the floor.

A similar pattern can be seen when a discus thrower starts to rotate in the ring (Figure 6.121). When both feet are in contact with the ground (right) and the force from the outer foot imparts rotation, both arms are outstretched to give the leg muscles time to act. When the thrower releases his foot, to put it in a new position for the second thrust, he pulls in the free arm towards his body to enable him to rotate quickly to get his foot down as fast as possible

and to gain balance, and to be able to generate force once again.

In most throws, rotation of the body starts with the help of one of the legs. The thrower gets into a position where the moment of inertia (*I*) is as large as possible (Figure 6.122). This means that the free arm is remote from the body, as is the free leg sometimes, and the upper body can be away from the axis of rotation.

At the moment you let go of the object being thrown the free arm is pulled close to and in front of the body, the legs are moved closer to each other and you become straighter in the hip area to ensure the rotation is as great as possible.

When the gymnast, the springboard diver or the high jumper puts his foot down during his final step, he determines how he will move in the air. If the force at take-off passes behind the body, the rotation will be directed so that it produces a somersault forwards (Figure 6.123A).

If the body is positioned, in relation to the feet, as shown in Figure 6.123B there will be a rotation backwards.

If you do not have the aid of external forces to create a rotation, it is possible to rotate a part of your body by a counter movement. A kick in soccer is most often finished in a position where you can obviously see how both arms and the upper body have rotated in the opposite direction to the kicking leg. To be able to keep good balance after the kick the angular momentum (*I* × ω) for the

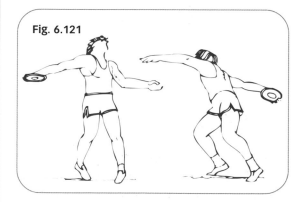

Fig. 6.121

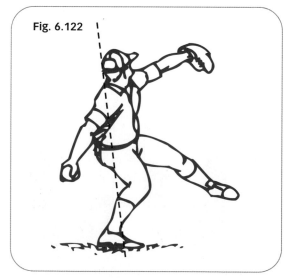

Fig. 6.122

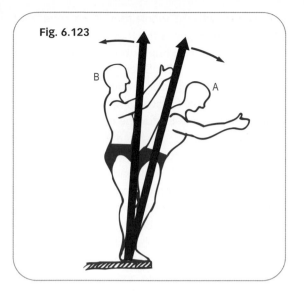

Fig. 6.123

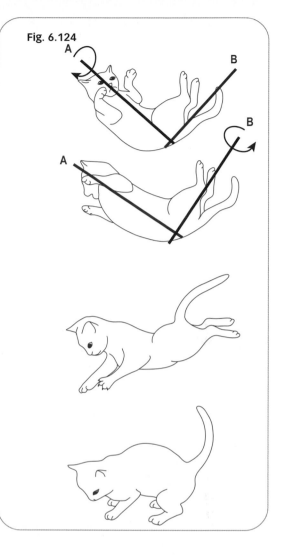

Fig. 6.124

upper body must equal the angular momentum ($I \times \omega$) for the kicking leg. Examples of counter-movements are described on pages 159–161.

We will look at the meaning of the expression:

Angular momentum (H) is constant if no external forces are acting.

This means that:

(I) If $H = 0$ you cannot create any angular momentum without access to external forces. If you jump up in the air without utilizing any external forces at all you cannot start a somersault or a twist in the air.
(II) If $H = 0$, changes in the body position can only be made by a counter-movement. One part of the body moves in one direction and another part moves in the opposite direction.
(III) If you have angular momentum after the take-off you cannot decrease or increase it in the air. It remains constant.
(IV) If you have angular momentum (for example, doing a somersault) you can 'steal' from this and produce a twist (rotation in another direction) but never increase or decrease the amount of angular momentum.

The cat in Figure 6.124 can be used to clarify the statements (I)–(IV).

How can a cat, which does not have any rotation at the beginning of a fall, twist in the air?

As we all know, a cat can do this very easily.

This is how it is done.

The cat takes up a position wherein the upper body makes an angle of 90° against the lower body. The forelegs are held close to the body and the hind legs are stretched out backwards as far as possible. The cat, which is very agile, can now rotate the upper body approximately 200° in the desired direction. The muscles that make this happen pull the lower body, at the same time, approximately 20° in the opposite direction. That the second rotation is much smaller depends on the fact that the moment of inertia of the lower body against the rotation around the A-axis is much larger (by a factor of 10 in the example) than for the lower body.

Now it is time for our feline friend to hold the forelegs away from the body and start to turn the lower body along the B-axis. The twist through 200° gives a counter-rotation of 20° on the lower body, which is now the most inert rotating part.

In the final position, the cat has turned through 180°. If the cat deems the rotation has not been fully carried through, it can rectify this by spinning its tail in a suitable direction. Half a turn with the tail sticking out perpendicularly from the body, could, at a guess, confer some 10° of counter-rotation to the body.

VII. Applications

This chapter concludes with the analysis of athletic performance utilizing anatomy and the laws of mechanics. On the basis of such an analysis, strength and flexibility training should be designed to suit the particular needs of the individual athlete. The sports technique we will examine here as an illustration is the long jump (Figures 6.125–6.132). We will consider in sequence: (a) run-up, (b) take-off, (c) flight and (d) landing. For each we will determine which muscles are active and how they operate (concentrically, eccentrically, statically). We will also determine which muscles require a wide range of movement, i.e. ought to be trained for flexibility.

(a) Run-up

Look at the way your foot strikes the ground. To minimize the risk of injury, the outer border of your foot should be the first part to make contact with the ground. Make sure your foot is pointing straight ahead of you, in the direction in which you are running. In general, striking the ground with the whole foot or with the front of the foot first, while the foot is pointed slightly outwards, leads to complaints of pain in the lower leg (periostitis, p. 77). Strong knee extensors – quadriceps femoris (four-headed thigh muscle, p. 65) – are essential for swinging the leg forward in running but, above all, for the correct heel strike. In the swing phase, the hip extensors – gluteus maximus (large buttock muscle) and hamstrings – should be sufficiently long and relaxed that they do not prevent a proper forward swing, i.e. hip flexion with the pelvis thrust forwards. During the forward thrust the body is supported by the forefoot of the stance-phase foot; therefore the triceps surae (three-headed calf muscle, p. 72) must be strong enough to prevent the body sinking 'backwards' at the ankle while the knee and hip extensors operate. The triceps surae operate statically during part of the stance phase, and concentrically in the later stages (Figure 6.126A and B).

The heel should be pulled towards the buttocks as early as possible, (i.e. concentric work for the knee flexors (hamstrings, p. 69) during the swing phase. This also provides flexibility training for the knee extensors (quadriceps, p. 65) and keeps the moment of inertia of the leg to a minimum during its forward swing. Thus, the speed of the forward swing is dependent on the strength of the hip flexors and the knee flexors, as well as the flexibility of the knee extensors. According to the above, training ought to concentrate on: (1), strengthening the iliopsoas, hamstrings, quadriceps and triceps surae, and (2), stretching the iliopsoas and quadriceps.

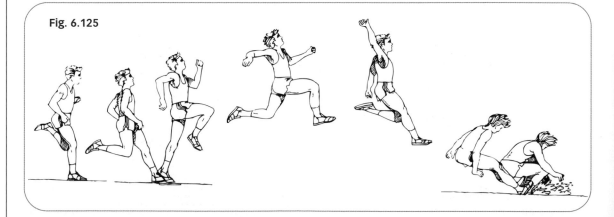

Fig. 6.125

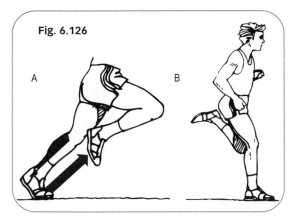

Fig. 6.126

A   B

(b) Take-off

At take-off the body has maximal speed. For a body travelling at a speed to reach as far as possible in a long jump, its angle of take-off should theoretically be about 45° (Figure 6.127). In practice, however, the jumper must hold back, i.e. steal some of his approach speed, in order to project himself upwards. To achieve a take-off angle of 45°, the force marshalled for upward thrust must be so great and directed so far back that speed after take-off is compromised and too low. The key to taking-off effectively thus lies in obtaining sufficient height without losing too much horizontal velocity.

Theoretically, a jumper can take off without reducing his speed only if the force of take-off is directed straight upwards. This would require a lightning swift upward thrust from a low position.

In some take-off styles the jumper takes a long third last stride and in so doing lowers his centre of gravity. By making the final stride relatively short, he is able to plant his lift-off foot on the ground more or less vertically from above (Figure 6.128). Even from a position that is as low as that, there is a possibility of effectively projecting the body upwards and forwards.

Attempts to obtain height in this way – without losing speed – result in take-off angles of about 20–25° and a reduction in speed of about 30%. This style requires an explosive forward thrust of the hip, knee and ankle (Figure 6.129).

The jumper may also obtain height by making a long final stride (Figure 6.130) and keeping his lift-off leg straighter than in the style outlined above. Take-off involves a greater contribution from hip extensor muscles (buttock muscles, p. 54) than from knee extensors.

These styles of take-off in the long jump can be contrasted with the high-jump styles, dive

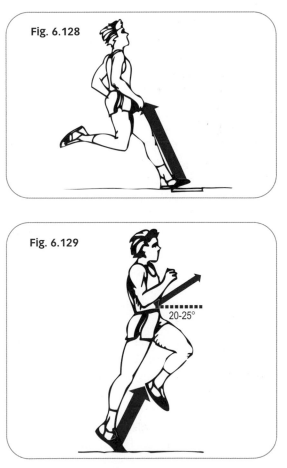

Fig. 6.128

Fig. 6.129

20-25°

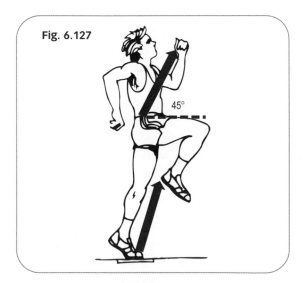

Fig. 6.127

45°

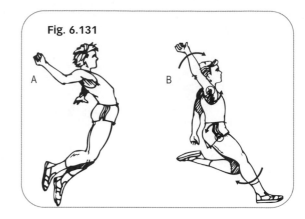

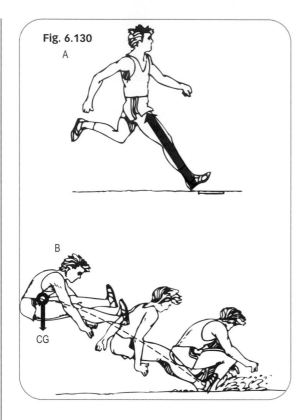

Fig. 6.130

A

B

CG

Fig. 6.131

A

B

straddle (deep knee flexion and emphasized free arm and leg movements) and Fosbury flop (greater speed of approach and bracing of the lift-off leg as strength of the hip is essential here).

We could also make comparisons between take-off styles in such sports as volleyball, football (to head the ball) and the like, when taking note of the speed of approach, i.e. the take-off styles requiring high-approach speed compared with those requiring low-approach speed.

(c) Flight

Whatever the take-off style, the jumper usually has a certain forward rotation. This rotation can be cancelled by adopting certain in-the-air techniques (Figure 6.131) such as (A) hang or (B) hitch-kick.

(Figure 6.131A.) If the jumper has a large forward rotation, he must lie outstretched in the air in order to avoid rotating so far that he arrives in an unfavourable position for landing. The speed of rotation is controlled by the body's moment of inertia (p. 169). The more he folds together, the greater (faster) will be his rotation. The less

rotation the jumper acquires from take-off, the sooner he can adopt a position that is advantageous for minimizing air resistance.

(Figure 6.131B.) If the rotation is too great, it must be countered by an opposing movement, i.e. the arms and legs should rotate in the same direction. If the arms move as indicated by the arrow, the body will move in the opposite direction at the shoulder joint, i.e. forward rotation is cancelled. A backward rotation of the legs as indicated by the arrow causes the pelvis to tilt in the other direction at the hip joint, i.e. forward rotation is cancelled.

(d) Landing

Landing requires good flexibility of the hamstrings and of the lower back. A maximal hip-piking before touchdown requires the action of the long muscles at the back of the thigh in order to avoid striking the ground with the heels too soon.

Maximal jump length is obtained when the heels touchdown at the point where the centre of gravity of the body would have landed (Figure 6.130B).

If the heel strike is too far in front of this point, the jumper will land on his buttocks. If his heels touch down too close to the take-off board, he will be seen to roll forwards at touchdown and, of course, the result will be poor.

In a perfect landing, the jumper is squeezed like an accordion, which subjects his knees to great stress. Therefore, his training must include deep knee flexion in order to prevent acute injuries.

Chapter 7

Hints for stretching

Examples of strength development and stretching exercises for different muscle groups accompany each section of the book, each of which describes a part of the body. The following diagrams summarize and complement these examples with positions that are designed to lengthen muscles and thereby increase the range of movement of a given body part. Sometimes several different positions are given for the same muscle group. It is up to you to choose the position (positions) that is (are) best suited to your particular needs. If you are 'stiff', certain positions will be suitable, or if your body is already rather flexible others should be chosen. Test the methods to find those that best suit you. Some variations of stretching methods, namely, elastic stretching, stretching and the PNF (proprioceptive neuromuscular facilitation) method, have been described on pp. 31–34. It should be pointed out that all types of flexibility training aim at producing a more flexible body; i.e. reaching the outer limits of the body's range of movement is the ultimate goal. Stretching is excellent for restoring a shortened muscle (due to injury or incorrect training methods) to its normal length. When a muscle has regained its normal length, it can be 'taught' to function correctly by submitting it to flexibility training consisting of flexibility and elastic stretching exercises.

Dancers have trained flexibility with elastic stretching for centuries; they provide excellent proof that this method of training yields good results. It cannot be stressed too strongly that it is essential to warm up before undertaking intensive exercise. Although a person can raise the temperature of particular muscles by static contraction (which is a part of the PNF method), if he wants to raise his entire body temperature substantially and, at the same time, subject his joints to all-round stress, he should begin any athletic activity with a well-prepared running-gymnastics-programme.

Stretching exercises

1. Stretching exercises should be part of warming up. Do not be afraid to make easy elastic stretches towards the outer limits of your range of movement, after you have first stretched in the ordinary manner for about 30 seconds. Muscle spindles (p. 22) are sensitive to both position (length changes) and rate of stretching (elastic stretching); therefore muscles must become accustomed to moving towards the body's outer limits at a moderate speed.
2. Either stretching exercises or PNF exercises should be a part of special training sessions

where the aim is to increase the length of a particular muscle group. Once he has been given suitable instructions, the athlete ought to be able to conduct these training sessions himself during periods (three times a week to increase flexibility; once or twice a week to maintain it) that do not interfere with other training such as team practice.

3. Stretching should be practised after heavy training sessions in order to avoid stiffness, soreness and muscular aches the following day. In this situation, stretching has the effect of lightly massaging the muscles.

Keep the principal objective in mind: a more flexible body. Positions for stretching and elastic stretching exercises for muscles that pass over specific parts of the body are shown below.

The front of the ankle (extensors, see Figure 7.1 and p. 76).

Do you find it difficult to sit comfortably on your heels? If so, this is due to your knees. Therefore, you must not try to lower yourself by stretching elastically if your knees hurt!

Goal: stretched, or somewhat overstretched ankle.

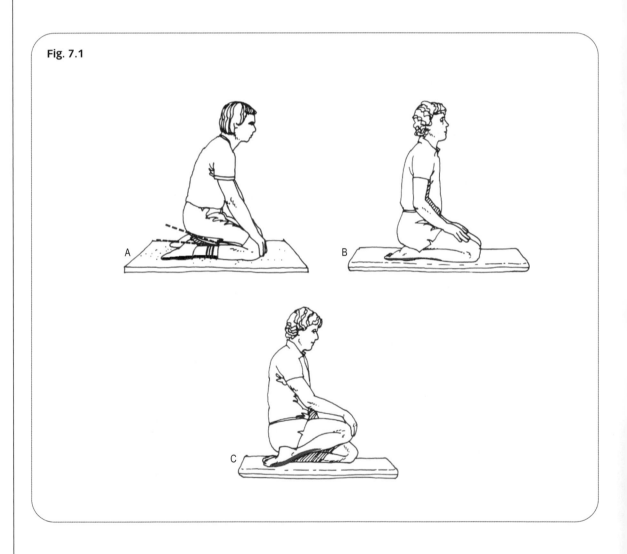

Fig. 7.1

Knee joint and back part of the hip (hamstrings, see Figure 7.4 and p. 69).

Goal: sufficient flexibility to allow a person to 'fall' forwards at the hip and not tax the back unnecessarily by 'bouncing'. Short muscles at the back of the thigh generally lead to lower back pain.

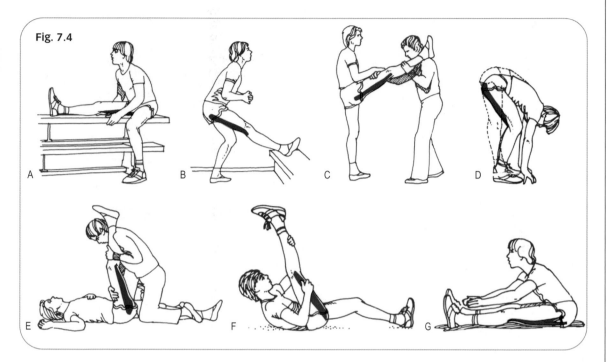

Fig. 7.4

Outer part of the hip (abductors, see Figure 7.5 and p. 54).

Goal: to increase flexibility of the hip and at the same time stretch the tendon band, which extends from the iliac crest (crest of the hip bone) down to the outer surface of the knee (iliotibial tract, see Figure 3.11). A tendon band that is too taut can lead to friction injuries of the lateral tibial condyle (external condyle of the shin bone) in, for example, the long distance runner (runner's knee).

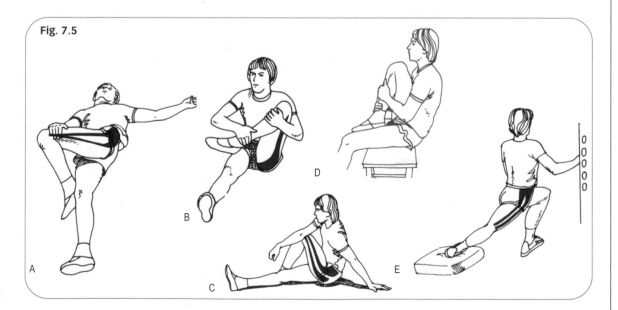

Fig. 7.5

Inner part of the hip (adductors, see Figure 7.6 and pp. 56–57).

Goal: increased flexibility for avoidance of groin injuries. Increased flexibility makes possible longer running strides, better forward push in ice-skating, longer stopping strides when attacking in badminton or tennis, etc.

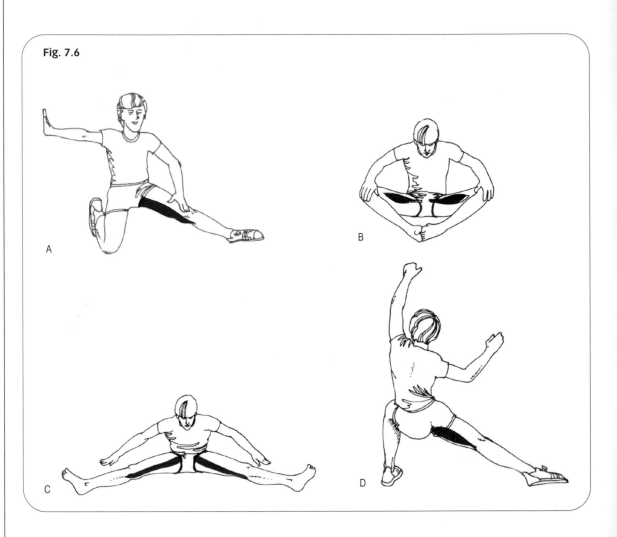

Fig. 7.6

A

B

C

D

Back and abdomen (erector spinae and abdominal muscles, pp. 94–100).
Goal: to increase flexibility of forward bending of the back. The diagrams (Figure 7.7) demonstrate positions that allow you to alternate between easy elastic stretching and relaxation.

The diagrams shown in Figure 7.8 demonstrate elastic stretching and positions suitable for sideward bending and rotation of the back.

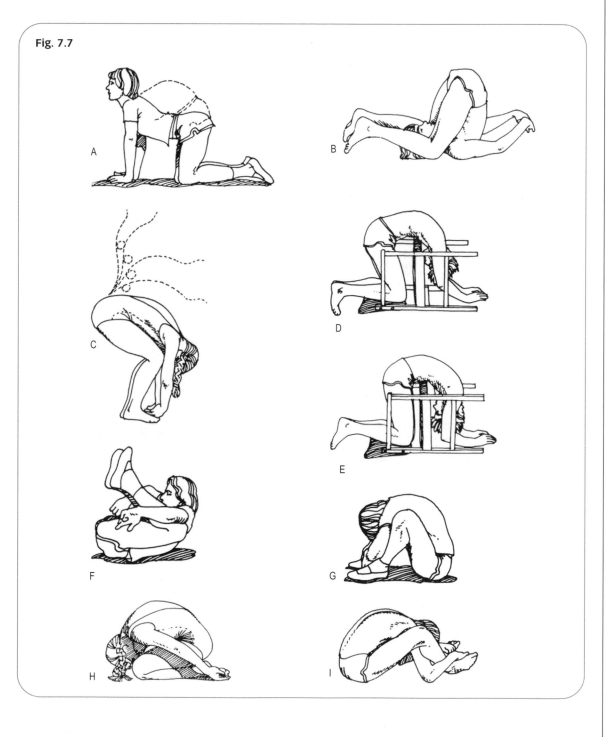

Fig. 7.7

Fig. 7.8

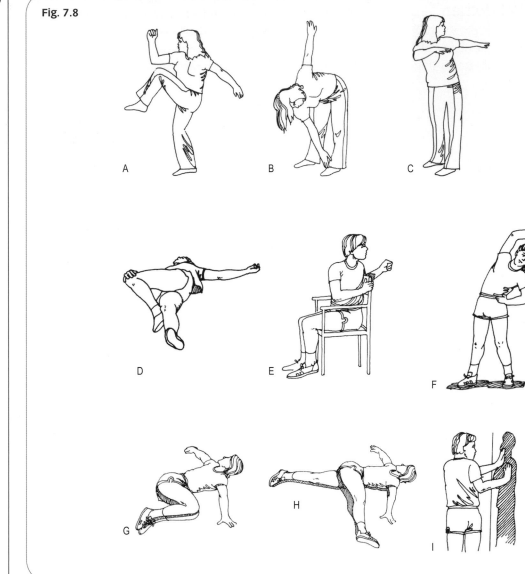

A

B

C

D

E

F

G

H

I

Shoulder joint (see Figure 7.9 and pp. 117–118).

Goal: increased flexibility of the shoulder which is often necessary in such sports as badminton, tennis, golf, handball and swimming.

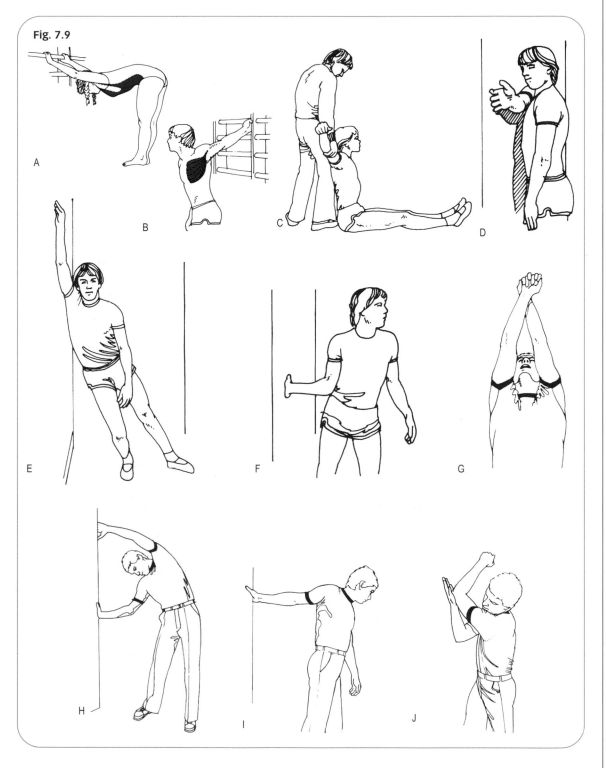

Fig. 7.9

Wrist (see Figures 7.10 and p. 127).

Goal: dorsiflexion flexibility. Applies to racket sports.

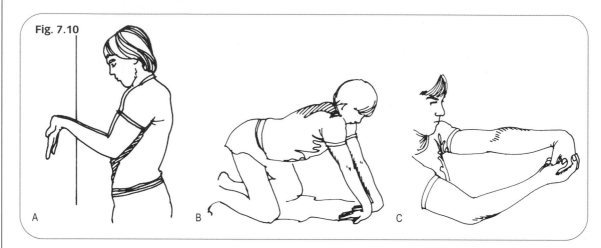

Fig. 7.10

A   B   C

Towel routine

It is easy to develop strength and flexibility by exercises with the aid of a towel. The four exercises shown in Figures 7.11–7.14 provide an example of how you can work dynamically with elastic stretches in order to increase the strength and flexibility of your shoulders.

The position in Exercise 3 is good for stretching the triceps brachii (three-headed arm muscle). There is seldom any need of stretching exercises for the muscles that pass over the elbow joint.

By using your imagination, you can easily develop your own exercises. It is a good idea to work in pairs. In that way you can both provide sufficient resistance to your partner in exercises that demand strength.

Exercise 1 (Figure 7.11). Keep the towel taut and 'dry' the back of your neck. Make sure that your grip is such that you can pull one of your arms with the other and thereby increase its flexibility a little bit each time. Repeat 20–30 times.

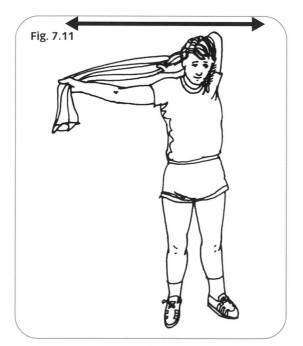

Fig. 7.11

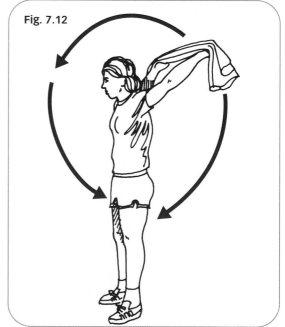

Fig. 7.12

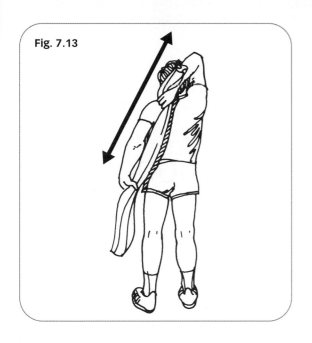

Fig. 7.13

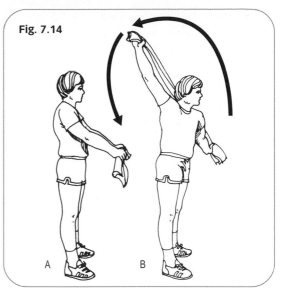

Fig. 7.14

Exercise 2 (Figure 7.12). Take hold of the towel in such a way that your hands are far enough apart to allow you to move both arms over your head as you alternate between lowering the towel in front of your thighs and behind them. Keep your arms straight and the towel taut. Move your arms closer to each other as you become more flexible. Do the exercise 20–30 times.

Exercise 3 (Figure 7.13). 'Dry your back'. Pull your right (bent) arm down with the aid of your left (straight) arm. After that, pull your straight arm up a little bit further with the aid of your bent arm. Do the exercise 10 times with bent right arm and 10 times with bent left arm.

Exercise 4 (Figure 7.14). (A) Hold the towel with your hands so far apart that you can (B) move the towel alternately in front of and behind your body with one straight arm at a time. In other words: a swimming action with 'backstrokes' takes the towel to the behind-your-back position, and with 'forward strokes', takes it to its original position. Do the exercise 20 times for each arm.

Review of relevant bones and muscles

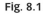

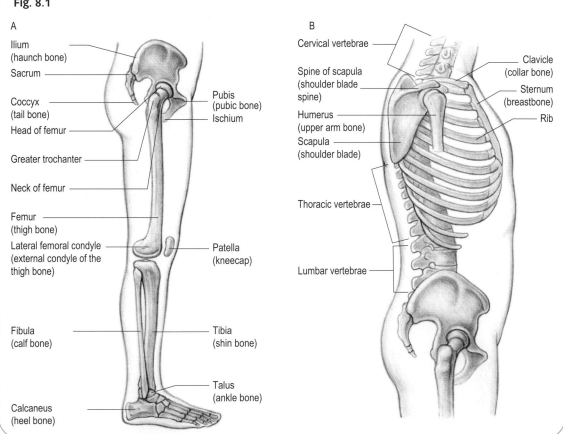

Chapter 8

Fig. 8.1

A

Ilium
(haunch bone)

Sacrum

Coccyx
(tail bone)

Head of femur

Greater trochanter

Neck of femur

Femur
(thigh bone)

Lateral femoral condyle
(external condyle of the
thigh bone)

Fibula
(calf bone)

Calcaneus
(heel bone)

Pubis
(pubic bone)

Ischium

Patella
(kneecap)

Tibia
(shin bone)

Talus
(ankle bone)

B

Cervical vertebrae

Spine of scapula
(shoulder blade
spine)

Humerus
(upper arm bone)

Scapula
(shoulder blade)

Thoracic vertebrae

Lumbar vertebrae

Clavicle
(collar bone)

Sternum
(breastbone)

Rib

Fig. 8.2

A

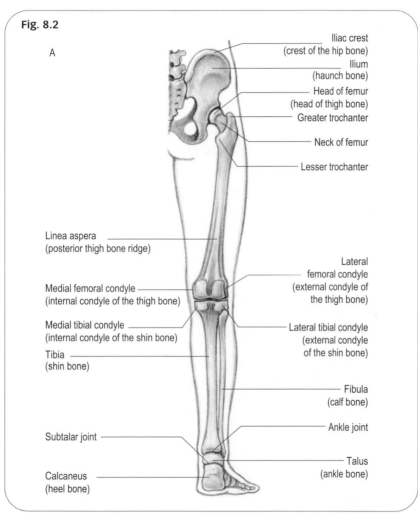

Iliac crest
(crest of the hip bone)

Ilium
(haunch bone)

Head of femur
(head of thigh bone)

Greater trochanter

Neck of femur

Lesser trochanter

Linea aspera
(posterior thigh bone ridge)

Lateral
femoral condyle
(external condyle of
the thigh bone)

Medial femoral condyle
(internal condyle of the thigh bone)

Medial tibial condyle
(internal condyle of the shin bone)

Lateral tibial condyle
(external condyle
of the shin bone)

Tibia
(shin bone)

Fibula
(calf bone)

Ankle joint

Subtalar joint

Talus
(ankle bone)

Calcaneus
(heel bone)

Continued

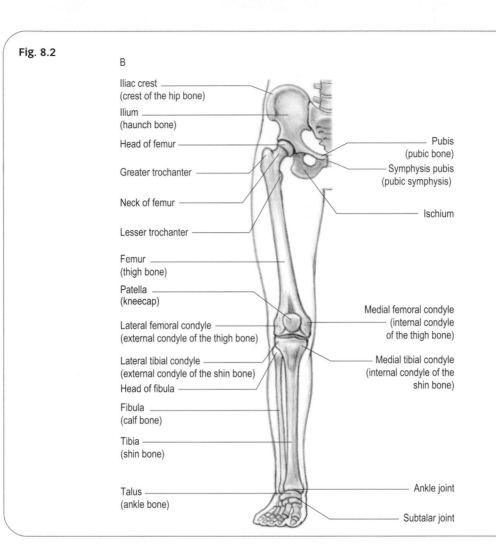

Fig. 8.2

B

Iliac crest
(crest of the hip bone)

Ilium
(haunch bone)

Head of femur

Greater trochanter

Neck of femur

Lesser trochanter

Femur
(thigh bone)

Patella
(kneecap)

Lateral femoral condyle
(external condyle of the thigh bone)

Lateral tibial condyle
(external condyle of the shin bone)

Head of fibula

Fibula
(calf bone)

Tibia
(shin bone)

Talus
(ankle bone)

Pubis
(pubic bone)

Symphysis pubis
(pubic symphysis)

Ischium

Medial femoral condyle
(internal condyle
of the thigh bone)

Medial tibial condyle
(internal condyle of the
shin bone)

Ankle joint

Subtalar joint

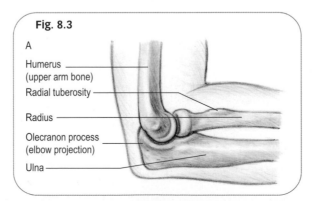

Fig. 8.3

A

Humerus
(upper arm bone)

Radial tuberosity

Radius

Olecranon process
(elbow projection)

Ulna

Continued

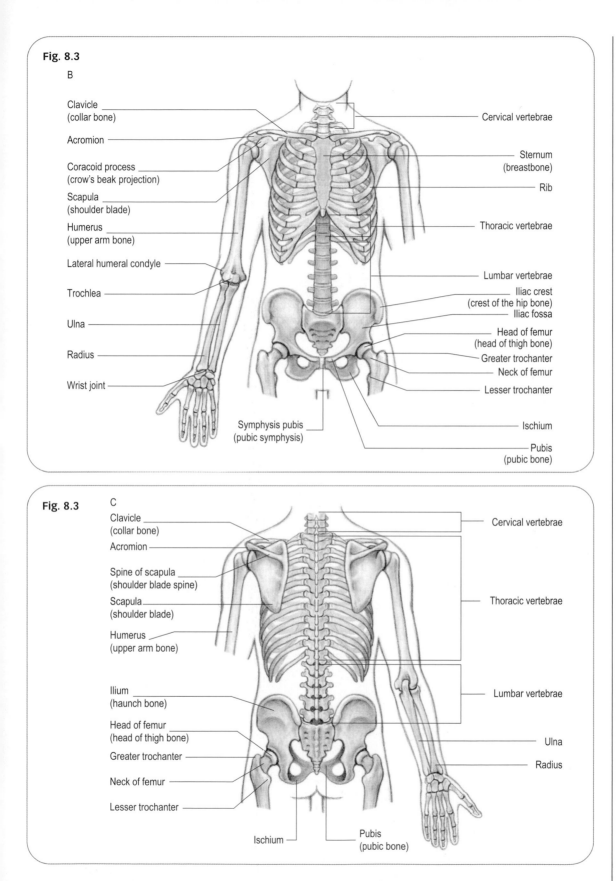

Fig. 8.3

B

- Clavicle (collar bone)
- Acromion
- Coracoid process (crow's beak projection)
- Scapula (shoulder blade)
- Humerus (upper arm bone)
- Lateral humeral condyle
- Trochlea
- Ulna
- Radius
- Wrist joint
- Symphysis pubis (pubic symphysis)

- Cervical vertebrae
- Sternum (breastbone)
- Rib
- Thoracic vertebrae
- Lumbar vertebrae
- Iliac crest (crest of the hip bone)
- Iliac fossa
- Head of femur (head of thigh bone)
- Greater trochanter
- Neck of femur
- Lesser trochanter
- Ischium
- Pubis (pubic bone)

Fig. 8.3

C

- Clavicle (collar bone)
- Acromion
- Spine of scapula (shoulder blade spine)
- Scapula (shoulder blade)
- Humerus (upper arm bone)
- Ilium (haunch bone)
- Head of femur (head of thigh bone)
- Greater trochanter
- Neck of femur
- Lesser trochanter
- Ischium
- Pubis (pubic bone)

- Cervical vertebrae
- Thoracic vertebrae
- Lumbar vertebrae
- Ulna
- Radius

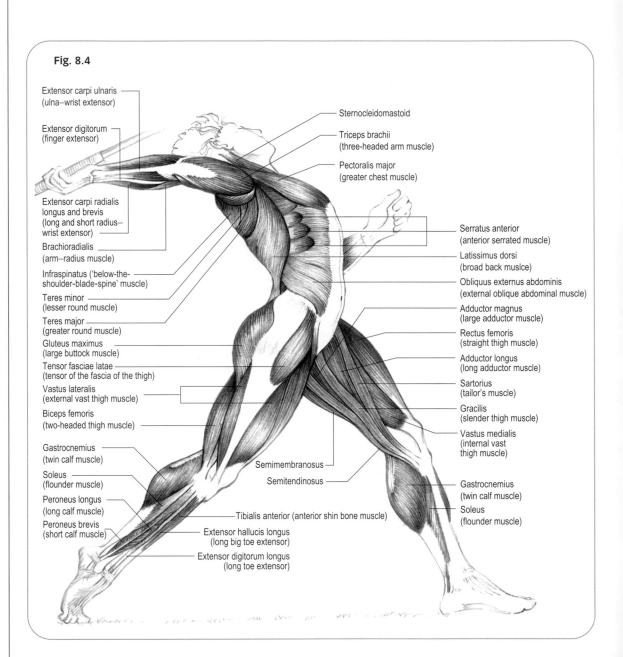

Fig. 8.4

Extensor carpi ulnaris
(ulna–wrist extensor)

Extensor digitorum
(finger extensor)

Extensor carpi radialis
longus and brevis
(long and short radius–
wrist extensor)

Brachioradialis
(arm–radius muscle)

Infraspinatus ('below-the-
shoulder-blade-spine' muscle)

Teres minor
(lesser round muscle)

Teres major
(greater round muscle)

Gluteus maximus
(large buttock muscle)

Tensor fasciae latae
(tensor of the fascia of the thigh)

Vastus lateralis
(external vast thigh muscle)

Biceps femoris
(two-headed thigh muscle)

Gastrocnemius
(twin calf muscle)

Soleus
(flounder muscle)

Peroneus longus
(long calf muscle)

Peroneus brevis
(short calf muscle)

Sternocleidomastoid

Triceps brachii
(three-headed arm muscle)

Pectoralis major
(greater chest muscle)

Serratus anterior
(anterior serrated muscle)

Latissimus dorsi
(broad back muslce)

Obliquus externus abdominis
(external oblique abdominal muscle)

Adductor magnus
(large adductor muscle)

Rectus femoris
(straight thigh muscle)

Adductor longus
(long adductor muscle)

Sartorius
(tailor's muscle)

Gracilis
(slender thigh muscle)

Vastus medialis
(internal vast
thigh muscle)

Gastrocnemius
(twin calf muscle)

Soleus
(flounder muscle)

Semimembranosus

Semitendinosus

Tibialis anterior (anterior shin bone muscle)

Extensor hallucis longus
(long big toe extensor)

Extensor digitorum longus
(long toe extensor)

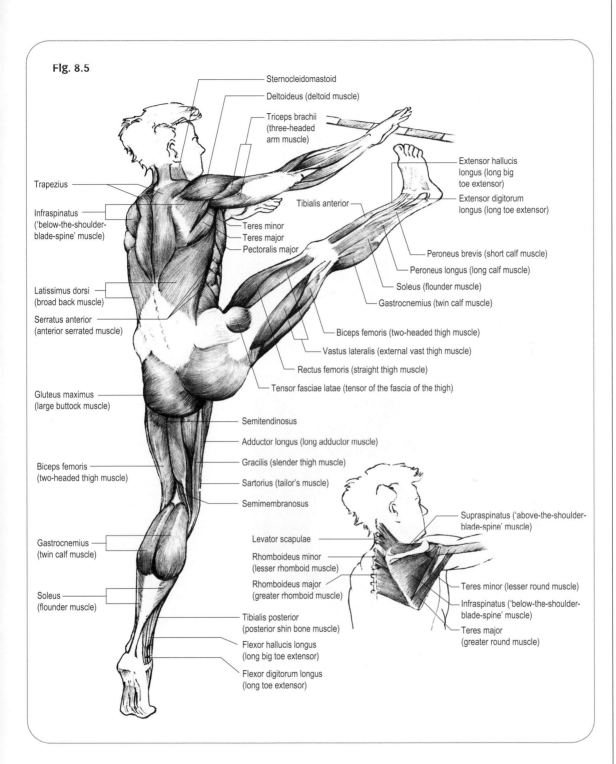

Fig. 8.5

Sternocleidomastoid

Deltoideus (deltoid muscle)

Triceps brachii (three-headed arm muscle)

Trapezius

Infraspinatus ('below-the-shoulder-blade-spine' muscle)

Latissimus dorsi (broad back muscle)

Serratus anterior (anterior serrated muscle)

Gluteus maximus (large buttock muscle)

Biceps femoris (two-headed thigh muscle)

Gastrocnemius (twin calf muscle)

Soleus (flounder muscle)

Teres minor
Teres major
Pectoralis major

Tibialis anterior

Extensor hallucis longus (long big toe extensor)

Extensor digitorum longus (long toe extensor)

Peroneus brevis (short calf muscle)

Peroneus longus (long calf muscle)

Soleus (flounder muscle)

Gastrocnemius (twin calf muscle)

Biceps femoris (two-headed thigh muscle)

Vastus lateralis (external vast thigh muscle)

Rectus femoris (straight thigh muscle)

Tensor fasciae latae (tensor of the fascia of the thigh)

Semitendinosus

Adductor longus (long adductor muscle)

Gracilis (slender thigh muscle)

Sartorius (tailor's muscle)

Semimembranosus

Levator scapulae

Rhomboideus minor (lesser rhomboid muscle)

Rhomboideus major (greater rhomboid muscle)

Tibialis posterior (posterior shin bone muscle)

Flexor hallucis longus (long big toe extensor)

Flexor digitorum longus (long toe extensor)

Supraspinatus ('above-the-shoulder-blade-spine' muscle)

Teres minor (lesser round muscle)

Infraspinatus ('below-the-shoulder-blade-spine' muscle)

Teres major (greater round muscle)

Fig. 8.6

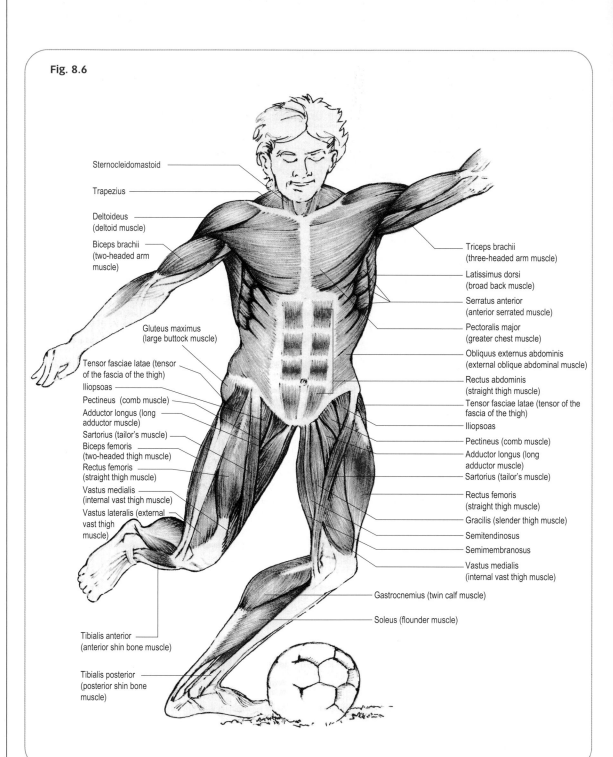

Sternocleidomastoid

Trapezius

Deltoideus
(deltoid muscle)

Biceps brachii
(two-headed arm
muscle)

Gluteus maximus
(large buttock muscle)

Tensor fasciae latae (tensor
of the fascia of the thigh)

Iliopsoas

Pectineus (comb muscle)

Adductor longus (long
adductor muscle)

Sartorius (tailor's muscle)

Biceps femoris
(two-headed thigh muscle)

Rectus femoris
(straight thigh muscle)

Vastus medialis
(internal vast thigh muscle)

Vastus lateralis (external
vast thigh
muscle)

Tibialis anterior
(anterior shin bone muscle)

Tibialis posterior
(posterior shin bone
muscle)

Triceps brachii
(three-headed arm muscle)

Latissimus dorsi
(broad back muscle)

Serratus anterior
(anterior serrated muscle)

Pectoralis major
(greater chest muscle)

Obliquus externus abdominis
(external oblique abdominal muscle)

Rectus abdominis
(straight thigh muscle)

Tensor fasciae latae (tensor of the
fascia of the thigh)

Iliopsoas

Pectineus (comb muscle)

Adductor longus (long
adductor muscle)

Sartorius (tailor's muscle)

Rectus femoris
(straight thigh muscle)

Gracilis (slender thigh muscle)

Semitendinosus

Semimembranosus

Vastus medialis
(internal vast thigh muscle)

Gastrocnemius (twin calf muscle)

Soleus (flounder muscle)

Tables of the body's most important muscles are presented in this chapter, together with their origin, insertion and function. In the following diagrams, origins and insertions of muscles are marked.

Muscles that pass across the hip joint only (pp. 54–58)

Muscle	Origin	Insertion	Function
Gluteus maximus (large buttock muscle)	Posterior part of the iliac crest (crest of the hip bone) the sacrum and coccyx (tail bone)	Outer surface of the femur (thigh bone) just below the greater trochanter and the iliotibial tract (a strong tendon band on the fascia of the thigh)	Straightens and adducts the hip, rotates the thigh out wards, and takes part in straightening the knee
Gluteus medius (intermediate buttock muscle)	Outer surface of the ilium	Greater trochanter of the femur	Primarily an abductor and inward rotator of the hip
Gluteus minimus (small buttock muscle)	Outer surface of the ilium immediately beneath and behind the gluteus medius	Greater trochanter of the femur	Same as the gluteus medius. Both are active during walking, and both stabilize the pelvis
Pectineus (comb muscle)	Upper border of the pubis (pubic bone)	High on the posterior surface of the femur (pectineal line)	Adducts and flexes the hip and rotates it outwards
Adductor brevis (short adductor muscle)	Lower border of the pubis	Linea aspera (posterior thigh bone ridge)	Adducts the hip and rotates it outwards
Adductor longus (long adductor muscle)	Near the symphysis pubis (pubic symphysis)	Linea aspera	Adducts the hip
Adductor magnus (large adductor muscle)	Two parts. One from the pubis and the other from the ischial tuberosity	Linea aspera and the medial (internal) femoral condyle	Adducts the hip. Can also rotate it inwards
Psoas major (great lumbar muscle)	Side of last thoracic vertebra (Th 12) and of lumbar vertebrae 1–4	These two muscles go under the common name of iliopsoas, which is attached to the lesser trochanter of the femur	Bends the hip. Rotates the leg outwards; can also bend the vertebral column sideways
Iliacus (haunch muscle)	Entire inner surface of the ilium		

Muscles that pass across both the hip and knee joints (pp. 61–70)

Muscle	Origin	Insertion	Function
Rectus femoris (straight thigh muscle)	Anterior inferior iliac spine and margin of the acetabulum (cotyloid cavity)	Patella (kneecap) via quadriceps femoris (four-headed thigh muscle) tendon	Straightens the knee and bends the hip
Gracilis (slender thigh muscle)	Pubis (pubic bone)	Pes anserinus (the 'goose foot' at the top of the inner surface of the tibia (shin bone))	Adducts the hip. Bends the knee and rotates it inwards
Tensor fasciae latae (tensor of the fascia of the thigh)	Outer surface of the spina iliaca anterior superior (anterior superior iliac spine)	Iliotibial tract (a strong tendon band on the fascia of the thigh)	Bends and abducts the hip and straightens the knee
Biceps femoris (two-headed thigh muscle)	Ischial tuberosity and linea aspera (posterior thigh bone ridge)	Head of the fibula (head of the calf bone)	Straightens (extends) the hip. Bends the knee and rotates it outwards
Semitendinosus	Ischial tuberosity	Pes anserinus	Straightens the hip. Bends the knee and rotates it inwards
Semimembranosus	Ischial tuberosity	Several sites on and around the medial (internal) tibial condyle	Straightens the hip. Bends the knee and rotates it inwards
Sartorius (tailor's muscle)	Spina iliaca anterior superior	Pes anserinus	Bends, abducts and rotates the hip outwards. Bends the knee and rotates it inwards

Muscles that pass across the knee joint only (p. 65)

Muscle	Origin	Insertion	Function
Vastus medialis (internal vast thigh muscle)	Medial (internal) and posterior surface of the femur (thigh bone)	Direct to the patella (kneecap)	Together with the rectus femoris (straight thigh muscle), these muscles form the quadriceps femoris (four-headed thigh muscle)
Vastus intermedius (central vast thigh muscle)	Anterior surface of the femur	Patella via the quadriceps tendon	The vasti muscles straighten the knee. The rectus femoris also bends the hip
Vastus lateralis (external vast thigh muscle)	Posterior surface of the femur	Patella via the quadriceps tendon	
Popliteus	Posterior surface of the lateral (external) femoral condyle	Posterior surface of the medial tibial condyle (internal condyle of the shin bone)	Bends the knee and rotates it inwards. ('Unlocks' the knee joint)

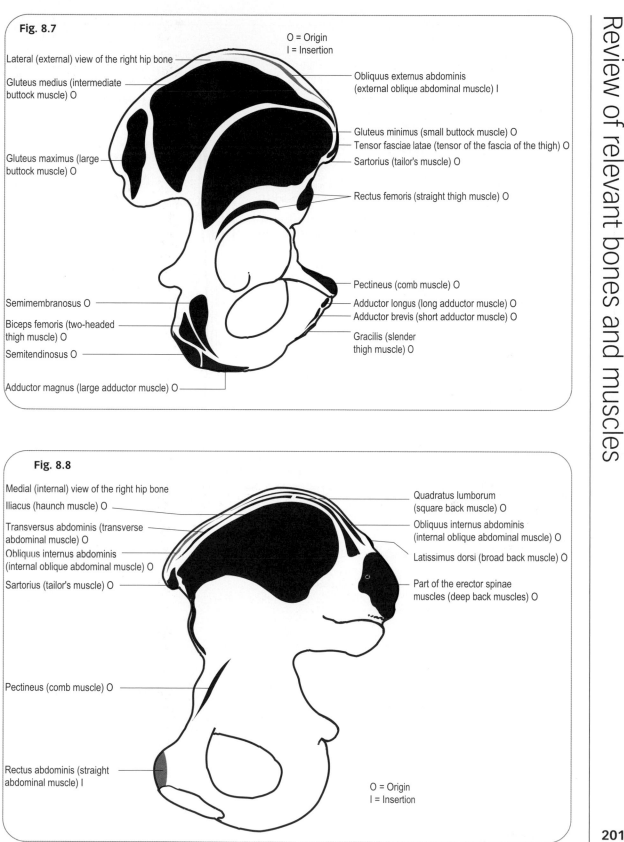

Fig. 8.7

O = Origin
I = Insertion

Lateral (external) view of the right hip bone

Gluteus medius (intermediate buttock muscle) O

Gluteus maximus (large buttock muscle) O

Semimembranosus O

Biceps femoris (two-headed thigh muscle) O

Semitendinosus O

Adductor magnus (large adductor muscle) O

Obliquus externus abdominis (external oblique abdominal muscle) I

Gluteus minimus (small buttock muscle) O
Tensor fasciae latae (tensor of the fascia of the thigh) O
Sartorius (tailor's muscle) O

Rectus femoris (straight thigh muscle) O

Pectineus (comb muscle) O
Adductor longus (long adductor muscle) O
Adductor brevis (short adductor muscle) O
Gracilis (slender thigh muscle) O

Fig. 8.8

Medial (internal) view of the right hip bone

Iliacus (haunch muscle) O

Transversus abdominis (transverse abdominal muscle) O

Obliquus internus abdominis (internal oblique abdominal muscle) O

Sartorius (tailor's muscle) O

Pectineus (comb muscle) O

Rectus abdominis (straight abdominal muscle) I

Quadratus lumborum (square back muscle) O

Obliquus internus abdominis (internal oblique abdominal muscle) O

Latissimus dorsi (broad back muscle) O

Part of the erector spinae muscles (deep back muscles) O

O = Origin
I = Insertion

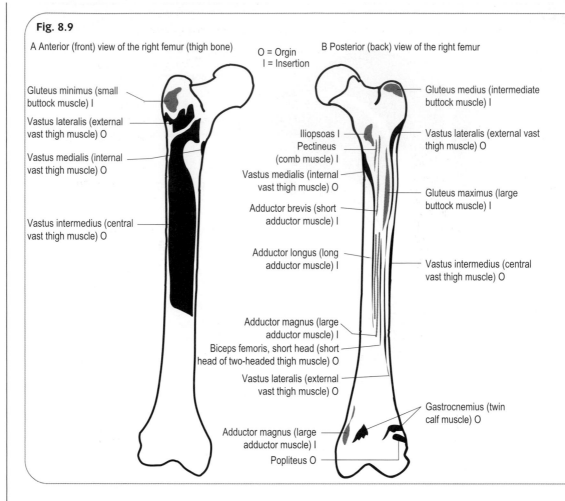

Fig. 8.9

A Anterior (front) view of the right femur (thigh bone)

O = Orgin
I = Insertion

B Posterior (back) view of the right femur

Gluteus minimus (small buttock muscle) I

Vastus lateralis (external vast thigh muscle) O

Vastus medialis (internal vast thigh muscle) O

Vastus intermedius (central vast thigh muscle) O

Iliopsoas I
Pectineus (comb muscle) I

Vastus medialis (internal vast thigh muscle) O

Adductor brevis (short adductor muscle) I

Adductor longus (long adductor muscle) I

Adductor magnus (large adductor muscle) I

Biceps femoris, short head (short head of two-headed thigh muscle) O

Vastus lateralis (external vast thigh muscle) O

Adductor magnus (large adductor muscle) I

Popliteus O

Gluteus medius (intermediate buttock muscle) I

Vastus lateralis (external vast thigh muscle) O

Gluteus maximus (large buttock muscle) I

Vastus intermedius (central vast thigh muscle) O

Gastrocnemius (twin calf muscle) O

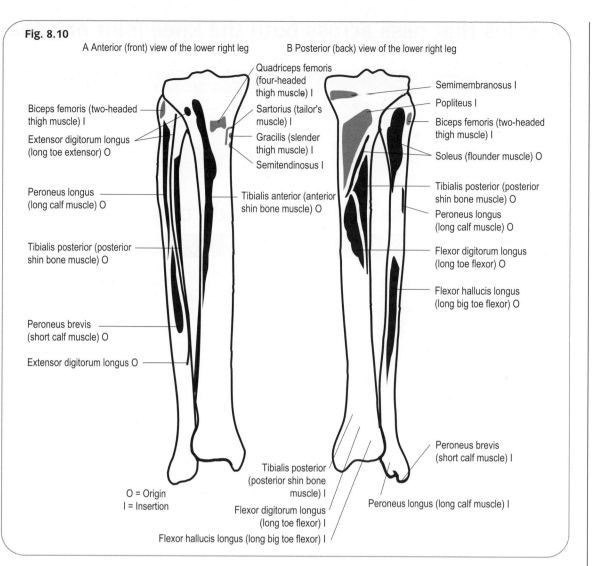

Fig. 8.10

A Anterior (front) view of the lower right leg

B Posterior (back) view of the lower right leg

Biceps femoris (two-headed thigh muscle) I

Extensor digitorum longus (long toe extensor) O

Peroneus longus (long calf muscle) O

Tibialis posterior (posterior shin bone muscle) O

Peroneus brevis (short calf muscle) O

Extensor digitorum longus O

Quadriceps femoris (four-headed thigh muscle) I

Sartorius (tailor's muscle) I

Gracilis (slender thigh muscle) I

Semitendinosus I

Tibialis anterior (anterior shin bone muscle) O

Semimembranosus I

Popliteus I

Biceps femoris (two-headed thigh muscle) I

Soleus (flounder muscle) O

Tibialis posterior (posterior shin bone muscle) O

Peroneus longus (long calf muscle) O

Flexor digitorum longus (long toe flexor) O

Flexor hallucis longus (long big toe flexor) O

Peroneus brevis (short calf muscle) I

Peroneus longus (long calf muscle) I

O = Origin
I = Insertion

Tibialis posterior (posterior shin bone muscle) I

Flexor digitorum longus (long toe flexor) I

Flexor hallucis longus (long big toe flexor) I

203

Muscles that pass across both the knee joint and the ankle (p. 72)

Muscle	Origin	Insertion	Function
Gastrocnemius (twin calf muscle)	Posterior surface of the medial and lateral femoral condyles (internal and external condyles of the thigh bone)	Calcaneus (heel bone)	Bends the knee and straightens the ankle (plantarflexion)

Muscles that pass across the ankle only (p. 76)

Muscle	Origin	Insertion	Function
Soleus (flounder muscle)	Head of the fibula (thigh bone) and from the oblique line of the tibia (shin bone)	Calcaneus (heel bone) Joins with the gastrocnemius (twin calf muscle) to form the triceps surae (three-headed calf muscle)	Standing on the toes (plantarflexion)
Tibialis anterior (anterior shin bone muscle)	Upper end of the tibia	Intermediate cuneiform (wedge-shaped) bone and the 1st metatarsal (bone of the foot)	Dorsiflexion and supination
Extensor hallucis longus (long big toe extensor)	Fibula and the interosseus membrane situated between the fibula and tibia	Big toe	Dorsiflexion and pronation of the ankle. Straightens the big toe and tibia
Extensor digitorum longus (long toe extensor)	Interosseus membrane between the fibula and tibia as well as the fascia of the lower legs	All the toes except the big toe	Dorsiflexion and pronation of the ankle. Stretches the toes
Peroneus longus (long calf muscle)	Upper part of the fibula	Its tendon of insertion passes behind the medial (external) malleolus, crosses the sole of the foot and is inserted into the big toe and the internal cuneiform bone	Builds up the transverse arch. Dorsiflexion and pronation of the ankle
Peroneus brevis (short calf muscle)	Lower part of the fibula	Fifth metatarsal	Dorsiflexion and pronation of the ankle
Flexor hallucis longus (long big toe flexor)	Posterior surface of the fibula	Underside of the big toe	Plantarflexion and supination. Bends the toes
Flexor digitorum longus (long toe flexor)	Posterior surface of the tibia	Underside of the toes (excepting the big toe)	Plantarflexion and supination. Bends the great toe
Tibialis posterior (posterior shin bone muscle)	Posterior surface of the fibula and tibia	Underside of the navicular (boat-shaped) bone	Plantarflexion and supination

Muscles whose origin is on the scapula (shoulder blade) and insertion on the humerus (upper arm bone) (pp. 112 and 113)

Muscle	Origin	Insertion	Function
Supraspinatus ('above-the-shoulder-blade-spine' muscle)	Fossa supraspinatus (an area above the shoulder blade spine)	Greater tuberosity of the humerus (upper arm bone)	Abducts and rotates the arm outwards
Teres major (greater round muscle)	Angulus inferior scapulae (inferior angle of the shoulder blade)	Medial lip of the intertubercular sulcus (internal lip of the biceps groove, on the anterior surface of the humerus)	Adducts the arm and rotates it inwards. (Assists the broad back muscle)
Infraspinatus ('below-the-shoulder-blade-spine' muscle)	A large part of the surface of the fossa infraspinata (an area underneath the shoulder blade spine)	Greater tuberosity of the humerus	Adducts and rotates the arm outwards
Teres minor (lesser round muscle)	Margo lateralis scapulae (outer border of the shoulder blade)	Greater tuberosity of the humerus	Adducts and rotates the arm outwards
Subscapularis (anterior shoulder blade muscle)	Fossa subscapularis (entire inner surface of the shoulder blade)	Lesser tuberosity of the humerus	Adducts and rotates the arm inwards
Coracobrachialis	Coracoid process (crow's beak projection)	Inner surface of the humerus	Swings the arm forwards

Muscles whose origin is on the trunk and insertion is on the scapula (shoulder blade) (p. 114)

Muscle	Origin	Insertion	Function
Levator scapulae	Cervical vertebrae 1–4	Angulus superior scapulae (superior angle of the shoulder blade)	Raises the scapula
Rhomboideus minor and major (lesser and greater rhomboid muscles)	Cervical vertebrae 6 and 7, thoracic vertebrae 1–4	Inner border of the scapula	Adducts the scapula and rotates it inwards
Trapezius	Base of the skull. Cervical and thoracic vertebrae	Scapula and external part of the clavicle (collar bone)	Adducts the scapula and rotates it outwards. Turns the head, bends the neck backwards
Serratus anterior (anterior serrated muscle)	Ribs 1–9	Inner border of the scapula	Stabilizes the scapula when the hand presses against an object
Pectoralis minor (lesser chest muscle)	Ribs 3–5	Coracoid process (crow's beak projection)	Lowers the scapula

Muscles whose origin is on the trunk and insertion is on the humerus (upper arm bone) (pp. 115–117)

Muscle	Origin	Insertion	Function
Pectoralis major (greater chest muscle)	Inner part of the clavicle (collar bone), sternum (breastbone), and part of the costal (rib) cartilage	Greater tuberosity of humerus and lateral lip of the intertubercular sulcus (external lip of the biceps groove)	Adducts the arm and rotates it inwards. Pulls the arm in front of the chest from any position
Deltoideus (deltoid muscle)	Outer part of the clavicle and the spine of scapula (shoulder blade spine)	Deltoid tuberosity (along the shaft of the upper arm bone)	Takes part in all movements of the upper arm
Latissimus dorsi (broad back muscle)	Dorsal vertebrae 6–12. Posterior part of the iliac crest (crest of the hip bone) and ribs 9–12. Rump bone	Floor of the intertubercular sulcus	Swings the arm backwards and rotates it inwards

Muscles that pass across both the shoulder and elbow joints (pp. 120–124)

Muscle	Origin	Insertion	Function
Biceps brachii (two-headed arm muscle)	(1) Coracoid process (crow's beak projection)	Radial tuberosity (on the anterior surface of the radius)	Bends and supinates the elbow.
	(2) Supraglenoid tubercle (upper rim of the scapula's (shoulder blade's) articular surface)	Is also connected to the ulna by way of a tendon band	Swing the shoulder joint forwards
Triceps brachii (three-headed arm muscle)	(1) Infraglenoid tubercle (below the scapula's articular surface) (2) Posterior surface of the humerus (upper arm bone) 3) Posterior surface of the humerus	Olecranon process (elbow projection) and joint capsule	Stretches the elbow and protects the shoulder joint by keeping the capsular ligament taut

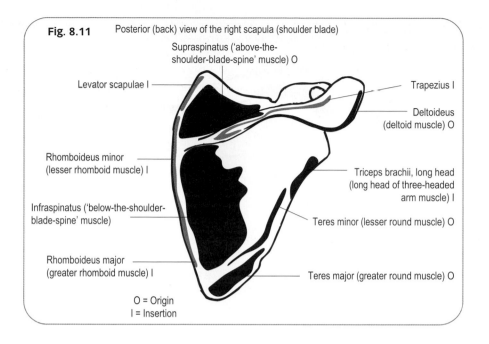

Fig. 8.11   Posterior (back) view of the right scapula (shoulder blade)

Supraspinatus ('above-the-shoulder-blade-spine' muscle) O

Levator scapulae I

Trapezius I

Deltoideus (deltoid muscle) O

Rhomboideus minor (lesser rhomboid muscle) I

Triceps brachii, long head (long head of three-headed arm muscle) I

Infraspinatus ('below-the-shoulder-blade-spine' muscle)

Teres minor (lesser round muscle) O

Rhomboideus major (greater rhomboid muscle) I

Teres major (greater round muscle) O

O = Origin
I = Insertion

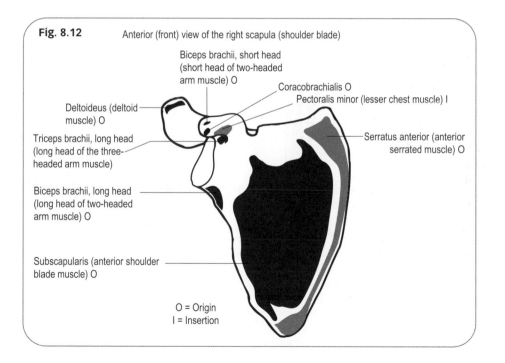

Fig. 8.12   Anterior (front) view of the right scapula (shoulder blade)

Biceps brachii, short head (short head of two-headed arm muscle) O

Coracobrachialis O

Pectoralis minor (lesser chest muscle) I

Deltoideus (deltoid muscle) O

Triceps brachii, long head (long head of the three-headed arm muscle)

Serratus anterior (anterior serrated muscle) O

Biceps brachii, long head (long head of two-headed arm muscle) O

Subscapularis (anterior shoulder blade muscle) O

O = Origin
I = Insertion

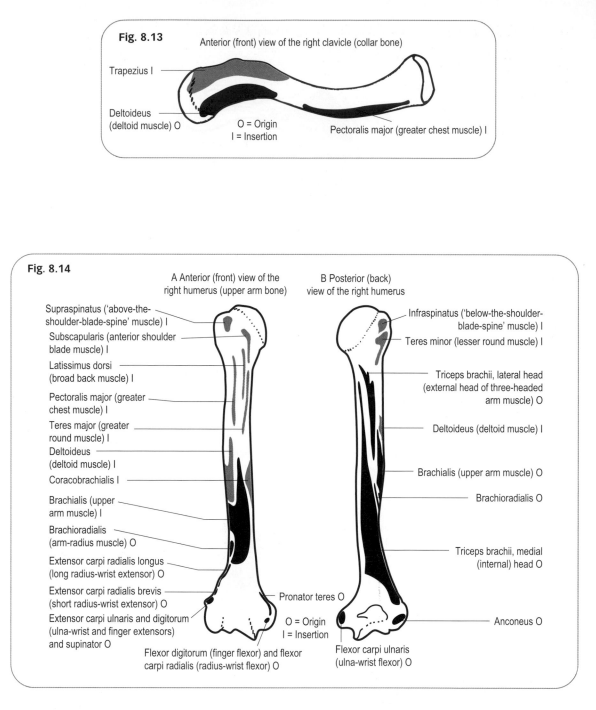

Fig. 8.13

Anterior (front) view of the right clavicle (collar bone)

Trapezius I

Deltoideus
(deltoid muscle) O

O = Origin
I = Insertion

Pectoralis major (greater chest muscle) I

Fig. 8.14

A Anterior (front) view of the
right humerus (upper arm bone)

B Posterior (back)
view of the right humerus

Supraspinatus ('above-the-
shoulder-blade-spine' muscle) I

Subscapularis (anterior shoulder
blade muscle) I

Latissimus dorsi
(broad back muscle) I

Pectoralis major (greater
chest muscle) I

Teres major (greater
round muscle) I

Deltoideus
(deltoid muscle) I

Coracobrachialis I

Brachialis (upper
arm muscle) I

Brachioradialis
(arm-radius muscle) O

Extensor carpi radialis longus
(long radius-wrist extensor) O

Extensor carpi radialis brevis
(short radius-wrist extensor) O

Extensor carpi ulnaris and digitorum
(ulna-wrist and finger extensors)
and supinator O

Pronator teres O

Flexor digitorum (finger flexor) and flexor
carpi radialis (radius-wrist flexor) O

O = Origin
I = Insertion

Infraspinatus ('below-the-shoulder-
blade-spine' muscle) I

Teres minor (lesser round muscle) I

Triceps brachii, lateral head
(external head of three-headed
arm muscle) O

Deltoideus (deltoid muscle) I

Brachialis (upper arm muscle) O

Brachioradialis O

Triceps brachii, medial
(internal) head O

Anconeus O

Flexor carpi ulnaris
(ulna-wrist flexor) O

Muscles that pass across the elbow joint only (pp. 120–123)

Muscle	Origin	Insertion	Function
Brachialis (upper arm muscle)	Greater part of the anterior surface of the humerus (upper arm bone)	Coronoid process (crown projection) of the ulna	Bends the elbow (flexes the forearm)
Brachioradialis (arm–radius muscle)		Styloid process of the radius	Bends the elbow (flexes the foream. Pronation or supination depending on the starting position
Anconeus	Posterior surface of the humerus	Posterior surface of the ulna	Straightens the elbow (extends the foream)
Supinator	Lateral (external) epicondyle of the humerus	Outer surface of the radius	Supinates the foream
Pronator teres	Medial (internal) epicondyle of the humerus	Outer surface of the radius	Pronates the forearm

Muscles that affect both the forearm and wrist (pp. 125–128)

Muscle	Origin	Insertion	Function
Extensor digitorum (finger extensor)	Lateral (external) epicondyle of the humerus (upper arm bone)	Posterior surface of the phalanges (fingers of the bones) (excepting the thumb)	Straightens the fingers, the wrist and finally the elbow
Extensor carpi radialis longus and brevis (long and short radius–wrist extensors)	Lateral (external) epicondyle of the humerus	Posterior of bases of the 2nd and 3rd metacarpals (bones of the hand)	Associated with extension and abduction of the wrist joint
Extensor carpi ulnaris (ulna–wrist extensor)	Lateral (external) epicondyle of the humerus	Posterior surface of the 5th metacarpal	Associated with extension and adduction of the wrist
Flexor digitorum superficialis (superficial finger flexor)	Medial (internal) epicondyle of the humerus and coronoid process (crown projection, on the anterior surface of the ulna)	Middle row of the phalanges	Bends the elbow and fingers. Assists in flexing the wrist radius
Flexor carpi radialis (radius–wrist flexor)	Medial (internal) epicondyle of the humerus	Anterior surface of the 2nd and 3rd metacarpals	Bends the elbow. When acting alone it flexes the wrist. Can also assist in pronating the forearm and hand
Flexor carpi ulnaris (ulna–wrist flexor)	Medial (internal) epicondyle and the inner margin of the olecranon process (elbow projection)	Pisiform, (pea-shaped) bone, hamate (hook-shaped) bone and 5th metacarpal	When acting alone it flexes the wrist and, by continuing to contract, it bends the elbow

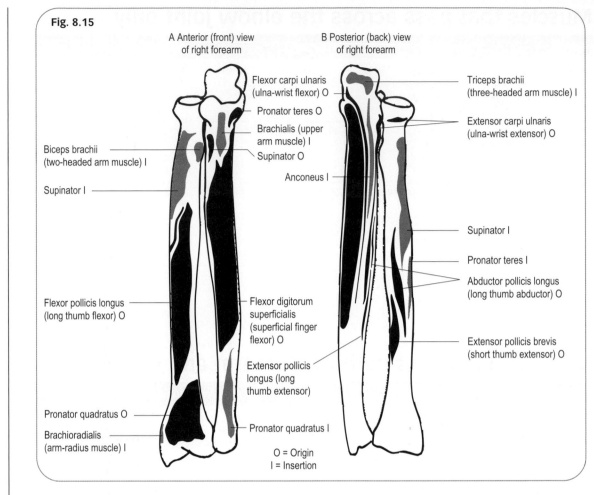

Fig. 8.15

A Anterior (front) view of right forearm

B Posterior (back) view of right forearm

Flexor carpi ulnaris (ulna-wrist flexor) O

Pronator teres O

Brachialis (upper arm muscle) I

Supinator O

Biceps brachii (two-headed arm muscle) I

Supinator I

Anconeus I

Triceps brachii (three-headed arm muscle) I

Extensor carpi ulnaris (ulna-wrist extensor) O

Supinator I

Pronator teres I

Abductor pollicis longus (long thumb abductor) O

Flexor pollicis longus (long thumb flexor) O

Flexor digitorum superficialis (superficial finger flexor) O

Extensor pollicis longus (long thumb extensor)

Extensor pollicis brevis (short thumb extensor) O

Pronator quadratus O

Pronator quadratus I

Brachioradialis (arm-radius muscle) I

O = Origin
I = Insertion

Index

Page numbers in italics refer to illustrations